THE ESSENCE OF MULTIVARIATE THINKING

Basic Themes and Methods

Multivariate Applications Series

Sponsored by the Society of Multivariate Experimental Psychology, the goal of this series is to apply complex statistical methods to significant social or behavioral issues, in such a way so as to be accessible to a nontechnical-oriented readership (e.g., nonmethodological researchers, teachers, students, government personnel, practitioners, and other professionals). Applications from a variety of disciplines, such as psychology, public health, sociology, education, and business, are welcome. Books can be single- or multiple-authored, or edited volumes that: (1) demonstrate the application of a variety of multivariate methods to a single, major area of research; (2) describe a multivariate procedure or framework that could be applied to a number of research areas; or (3) present a variety of perspectives on a controversial topic of interest to applied multivariate researchers.

There are currently nine books in the series:

- *What if there were no significance tests?* co-edited by Lisa L. Harlow, Stanley A. Mulaik, and James H. Steiger (1997).
- *Structural Equation Modeling with LISREL, PRELIS, and SIMPLIS: Basic Concepts, Applications, and Programming* written by Barbara M. Byrne (1998).
- *Multivariate Applications in Substance Use Research: New Methods for New Questions,* co-edited by: Jennifer S. Rose, Laurie Chassin, Clark C. Presson, and Steven J. Sherman (2000).
- *Item Response Theory for Psychologists*, co-authored by Susan E. Embretson and Steven P. Reise (2000).
- *Structural Equation Modeling with AMOS: Basic Concepts, Applications, and Programming*, written by Barbara M. Byrne (2001).
- *Conducting Meta-Analysis Using SAS*, written by Winfred Arthur, Jr., Winston Bennett, Jr., and Allen I. Huffcutt (2001).
- *Modeling Intraindividual Variability with Repeated Measures Data: Methods and Applications*, co-edited by D. S. Moskowitz and Scott L. Hershberger (2002).
- *Multilevel Modeling: Methodological Advances, Issues, and Applications*, co-edited by Steven P. Reise and Naihua Duan (2003).
- *The Essence of Multivariate Thinking: Basic Themes and Methods* by Lisa Harlow (2005).

Anyone wishing to submit a book proposal should send the following: (1) author/title, (2) timeline including completion date, (3) brief overview of the book's focus, including table of contents, and ideally a sample chapter (or more), (4) a brief description of competing publications, and (5) targeted audiences.

For more information please contact the series editor, Lisa Harlow, at: Department of Psychology, University of Rhode Island, 10 Chafee Road, Suite 8, Kingston, RI 02881-0808; Phone: (401) 874-4242; Fax: (401) 874-5562; or e-mail: LHarlow@uri.edu. Information may also be obtained from members of the advisory board: Leona Aiken (Arizona State University), Gwyneth Boodoo (Educational Testing Service), Barbara M. Byrne (University of Ottawa), Patrick Curran (University of North Carolina), Scott E. Maxwell (University of Notre Dame), David Rindskopf (City University of New York), Liora Schmelkin (Hofstra University) and Stephen West (Arizona State University).

THE ESSENCE OF MULTIVARIATE THINKING

Basic Themes and Methods

Lisa L. Harlow
University of Rhode Island

LEA

2005

LAWRENCE ERLBAUM ASSOCIATES, PUBLISHERS

Mahwah, New Jersey London

Senior Editor:	Debra Riegert
Editorial Assistant:	Kerry Breen
Cover Design:	Kathryn Houghtaling Lacey and Lisa L. Harlow
Textbook Production Manager:	Paul Smolenski
Full-Service Compositor:	TechBooks
Text and Cover Printer:	Hamilton Printing Company

This book was typeset in 10/12 pt. Times, Italic, Bold, and Bold Italic. The heads were typeset in Americana, Americana Italic, and Americana Bold.

Lawrence Erlbaum Associates, Inc., Publishers
10 Industrial Avenue
Mahwah, New Jersey 07430
www.erlbaum.com

Library of Congress Cataloging-in-Publication Data

Harlow, Lisa Lavoie, 1951–
    The essence of multivariate thinking : basic themes and methods / Lisa L. Harlow.
        p. cm.—(Multivariate applications book series)
    Includes bibliographical references and index.
    ISBN 0-8058-3729-9 (hardback : alk. paper)—ISBN 0-8058-3730-2 (pbk. : alk. paper)
    1. Multivariate analysis. 2. Psychology—Mathematical models.   I. Title.   II. Series.

    QA278.H349 2005
    519.5'35—dc22   2004028095

Books published by Lawrence Erlbaum Associates are printed on acid-free paper, and their bindings are chosen for strength and durability.

Printed in the United States of America
10 9 8 7 6 5 4 3 2 1

*In memory of
Jacob Cohen*

Contents

IV: MULTIVARIATE GROUP METHODS

List of Figures and Tables

Figures

Tables

Preface

The current volume was written with a simple goal: to make the topic of multivariate statistics more accessible and comprehensible to a wide audience. To encourage a more encompassing cognizance of the nature of multivariate methods, I suggest basic themes that run through most statistical methodology. I then show how these themes are applied to several multivariate methods that could be covered in a statistics course for first-year graduate students or advanced undergraduates. I hope awareness of these common themes will engender more ease in understanding the basic concepts integral to multivariate thinking. In keeping with a conceptual focus, I kept formulas at a minimum so that the book does *not* require knowledge of advanced mathematical methods beyond basic algebra and finite mathematics. There are a number of excellent statistical works that present greater mathematical and statistical details than the current volume or present other approaches to multivariate methods. When possible I suggest references to some of these sources for those individuals who are interested.

Before delineating the content of the chapters, it is important to consider what prerequisite information would be helpful to have before studying multivariate methods. I recommend having a preliminary knowledge of basic statistics and research methods as taught at the undergraduate level in most social science fields. This foundation would include familiarity with descriptive and inferential statistics, the concepts and logic of hypothesis testing procedures, and effect sizes. Some discussion of these topics is provided later in this book, particularly as they relate to multivariate methods. I invite the reader to review the suggested or similar material to ensure good preparation at the introductory level, hopefully making an excursion into multivariate thinking more enjoyable.

CONTENTS

The first three chapters provide an overview of the concepts and approach addressed in this book. In Chapter 1, I provide an introductory framework for multivariate thinking and discuss benefits and drawbacks to using multivariate methods before providing a context for engaging in multivariate research.

In Chapter 2, I show how a compendium of multivariate methods is much more attainable if we notice several themes that seem to underlie these statistical techniques. These themes are elaborated to provide an overarching sense of the capabilities and scope of these procedures. The pivotal and pervasive theme of multivariate methods is multiplicity: the focus on manifold sources in the development of a strong system of knowledge. Use of these methods acknowledges and encourages attention on multiple ways of investigating phenomena. We can do this by widening our lens to identify multiple and relevant theories, constructs, measures, samples, methods, and time points. Although no single study can possibly encompass the full breadth of multiple resources we identify, multivariate methods allow us to stretch our thinking to embrace a wider domain to examine than we otherwise might pursue. This broadening approach at multiple levels provides greater reliability and validity in our research.

After acknowledging the emphasis on multiple foci, we delve into several additional themes that reoccur and seem to anchor many of the multivariate methods. These themes draw on the central notions of variance, covariance, ratios of variances and/or covariances, and linear combinations, all of which contribute to a summary of shared variance among multiple variables.

We are then ready to address themes that help in evaluating and interpreting results from multivariate methods. For each method discussed, I encourage a macro-assessment that summarizes findings with both significance tests and effect sizes. Recognizing that significance tests provide only limited information (e.g., the probability that results are due to chance), I also provide information on the magnitude of research findings with effect sizes. Results are also evaluated from a micro-perspective to determine the specific, salient aspects of a significant effect, which often include information about means or weights for variables.

In Chapter 3, I delineate several background themes that pertain to both univariate and multivariate methods. This includes discussion about data, sample, measurement, variables, assumptions, and preliminary screening to prepare data for analysis.

After gaining insight into the core themes, I turn to an illustration of these themes as they apply to several multivariate methods. The selection of methods (i.e., multiple regression, analysis of covariance, multivariate analysis of variance, discriminant function analysis, logistic regression, canonical correlation, principal components, and factor analysis) is limited to a subset of multivariate procedures that have wide application and that readily elucidate the underlying multivariate themes presented here.

In Chapters 4 and 5, I feature the themes with the intermediate multivariate methods of multiple regression and analysis of covariance, respectively, that bridge well-known univariate methods (e.g., correlation and analysis of variance) with other multivariate methods discussed later.

In Chapter 6, I provide an overview of matrix notation and calculations, enough to help in understanding subsequent chapters.

In Chapters 7, 8, and 9, I then discuss how the themes pertain to the multivariate group methods of multivariate analysis of variance, discriminant function analysis, and logistic regression that each incorporate a major categorical, grouping variable (e.g., gender, treatment, qualitative or ordinal outcome).

In Chapters 10 and 11, respectively, I apply the themes to multivariate correlational methods that are used in an exploratory approach: canonical correlation and a combined focus on principal components analysis and factor analysis.

In Chapter 12, I present an integration of the themes across each of the selected multivariate methods. This summary includes several charts that list common themes and how they pertain to each of the methods discussed in this book. I hope readers will leave with greater awareness and understanding of the essence of multivariate methods and how they can illuminate our research and ultimately our thinking.

LEARNING TOOLS

A detailed example is provided for each method to delineate how the multivariate themes apply and to provide a clear understanding and interpretation of the findings. Results from statistical analysis software programs are presented in tables that for the most part mirror sections of the output files.

Supplemental information is provided in the accompanying CD, allowing several opportunities for understanding the material presented in each chapter. Data from 527 women at risk for HIV provide a set of variables, collected over three time points, to highlight the multivariate methods discussed in this book. The data were collected as part of a National Institute of Mental Health grant (Principal investigators L. L. Harlow, K. Quina, and P. J. Morokoff) to predict and prevent HIV risk in women. The same data set is used throughout the book to provide a uniform focus for examples. SAS computer program and output files are given corresponding to the applications in the chapters. This allows readers to verify how to set up and interpret the analyses delineated in the book. A separate set of homework exercises and lab guidelines provide additional examples of how to apply the methods. Instructors and students can work through these when they want to gain practice applying multivariate methods. Finally, lecture summaries are presented to illuminate the main points from the chapters.

ACKNOWLEDGMENTS

This book was partially supported by a Fulbright Award while I was at York University, Toronto, Ontario, Canada; by a National Science Foundation grant on multidisciplinary learning communities in science and engineering (Co-principal investigators: Donna Hughes, Lisa Harlow, Faye Boudreaux-Bartels, Bette Erickson, Joan Peckham, Mercedes Rivero-Herdec, Barbara Silver, Karen Stein, and Betty Young), and by a National Science Foundation grant on advancing women in the sciences, technology, engineering and mathematics (principal investigator: Janett Trubatch).

Thanks are offered to all the students, faculty, and staff at the University of Rhode Island, York University, and the Cancer Prevention Research Center who generously offered resources, support, and comments. I am deeply indebted to the many students I have taught over the years, who have raised meaningful questions and provided insightful comments to help clarify my thinking.

I owe much to the National Institute of Mental Health for a grant on prediction of HIV risk in women and to Patricia Morokoff and Kathryn Quina, my collaborators on the grant. Without the grant and the support of these incredible colleagues, the data, examples, and analyses in this book would not be possible.

Much recognition is extended to Tara Smith, Kate Cady-Webster, and Ana Bridges, all of whom served as teaching assistants and/or (co-)instructors of multivariate courses during the writing of this book. Each of these intelligent and dedicated women continually inspires me to greater clarity in my thinking. In particular, Tara helped me immeasurably in developing lab exercises, and Kate helped with some of the lecture summaries for the chapters. Their help made it possible for me to include a CD supplement for this text.

I am very grateful to Dale Pijanowski who generously shared her joyous and positive spirit about my writing at a time when I was not as convinced as she was that this book would be finished.

I owe many thanks to Barbara Byrne and Keith Markus, who provided detailed and constructive reviews of several preliminary chapters. Their thoughtful comments went a long way toward improving the book, but any remaining errors are most certainly my own.

Lawrence Erlbaum Associates—in particular, Debra Riegert and Larry Erlbaum—deserve my highest praise for unfailing support, encouragement, and a wealth of expertise. Nicole McClenic also gets a gold star as project manager.

Appreciation is offered to the Society of Multivariate Experimental Psychology (SMEP) that offers an ongoing forum in which to stay informed and enlightened in state-of-the-art methodology. I especially want to express my enduring gratitude for the wisdom that freely flowed and was generously bestowed on all SMEP members by Jacob (Jack) Cohen, whose memory permeates the hearts and minds of all of us fortunate enough to have been in his presence, if only much too briefly. Jack had a no-nonsense style that cut through all fuzziness and vagaries of thinking, all the while pleasantly illuminating key concepts with such erudite acumen that no one could leave him feeling uninformed. If ever there were a guru of pivotal statistical insight, it assuredly would be Jack.

Finally, my heartfelt thanks are extended to my husband, Gary, and daughter, Rebecca, who are a constant source of support and inspiration to me. Gary was also instrumental in providing extensive production assistance with formatting the text, tables, and the accompanying supplements in the CD. I consider myself very fortunate to have been gifted with my family's functional support as well as their unyielding tolerance of and encouragement to having me spread the word about the wonders and marvels of multivariate thinking.

I

Overview

1

Introduction

WHAT IS MULTIVARIATE THINKING?

In much of science and life, we often are trying to understand the underlying truth in a morass of observable reality. Herbert Simon (1969) states that we are attempting to find the basic simplicity in the overt complexity of life. Margaret Wheatley (1994), a social scientist working with organizations, suggests that we are seeking to uncover the latent order in a system while also recognizing that "It is hard to open ourselves to a world of inherent orderliness... trusting in the unfolding dance of order" (1994, p. 23). I would like to argue that the search for simplicity and latent order could be made much more attainable when approached with a mindset of multivariate thinking.

Multivariate thinking is defined as a body of thought processes that illuminate interrelatedness between and within sets of variables. The essence of multivariate thinking as portrayed in this book proposes to expose the inherent structure and to uncover the meaning revealed within these sets of variables through application and interpretation of various multivariate statistical methods with real-world data.

The multivariate methods we examine are a set of tools for analyzing multiple variables in an integrated and powerful way. The methods make it possible to examine richer and more realistic designs than can be assessed with traditional univariate methods that analyze only one outcome variable and usually just one or two independent variables. Compared with univariate methods, multivariate methods allow us to analyze a complex array of variables, providing greater assurance that we can come to some synthesizing conclusions with less error and more validity than if we were to analyze variables in isolation.

3

Multivariate knowledge offers greater flexibility and options for analyses that extend and enrich other statistical methods of which we have some familiarity. Ultimately, a study of multivariate thinking and methods encourages coherence and integration in research that hopefully can motivate policy and practice. A number of excellent resources exist for those interested in other approaches to multivariate methods (Cohen, Cohen, West, & Aiken, 2003; Gorsuch, 1999; Harris, 2001; Marcoulides & Hershberger, 1997; Tabachnick & Fidell, 2001).

Having a preliminary understanding of what is meant by multivariate thinking, it is useful to itemize several benefits and drawbacks to studying multivariate methods.

BENEFITS

Several benefits can be derived from understanding and using multivariate methods.

a. *First, our thinking is stretched to embrace a larger context in which we can envision more complex and realistic theories and models than could be rendered with univariate methods.* Knowledge of multivariate methods provides a structure and order with which to approach research, demystifying the aura of secrecy and laying bare the essence because most phenomena of interest to researchers are elaborate, involving several possible variables and patterns of relationship. We gain insight into methods that previously were perceived as abstract and incomprehensible by increasing our understanding of multivariate statistical terminology. The knowledge builds on itself, providing increased understanding of statistical methodology. Thus, multivariate thinking offers an intellectual exercise that expands our sense of knowing and discourages isolated, narrow perspectives. It helps sort out the seeming mystery in a research area, providing a large set of real-world approaches for analysis to explain variability in a nonconstant world.

b. *Second, a thorough grounding in multivariate thinking helps us understand others' research, giving us a richer understanding when reading the literature.* By studying the basic features and applications of these statistical tools, we can become better consumers of research, achieving greater comprehension of particular findings and their implications. Several students have reported that, whereas they previously had just scanned the abstracts and possibly the introduction and discussion sections of research articles, studying multivariate methods gave them the intellectual curiosity and the know-how to venture into the methods and results sections. Reading the statistical portion of research articles provided greater enjoyment when reading the literature and opened up a world replete with multiple approaches that can be applied to a research area. After continued exposure and experience with the many ways to apply multivariate methods, we can begin to develop a more realistic and critical view of others' research and gain more clarity on the merits of a body of research. Even if we never choose to conduct our own analyses, knowledge of multivariate methods opens our eyes to a wider body of research than would be possible with only univariate methods of study.

c. *Third, multivariate thinking helps expand our capabilities by informing application to our own research.* We are encouraged to consider multiple methods for our research, and the methods needed to perform research are more fully understood. An understanding of multivariate methods increases our ability to evaluate complex, real-world phenomena and encourages ideas on how to apply rigorous methods to our own research. Widening our lens to see more and own more information regarding research, we are encouraged to think in terms that lead to asking deeper, clearer, and richer questions. With this broadened perspective, we are able to see the connection between theory and statistical methods and potentially to inform theory development. Empirically, a background in multivariate methods allows us to crystallize theory into testable hypotheses and to provide empirical support for our observations. Thus, it can increase the credibility of our research and help us add to existing literature by informing an area with our unique input. We also are offered greater responsibility and are challenged to contribute to research and scholarly discourse in general, not exclusively in our own area of interest.

d. *Fourth, multivariate thinking enables researchers to examine large sets of variables in encompassing and integrated analysis, thereby controlling for overall error rate and also taking correlations among variables into account.* This is preferred to conducting a large number of univariate analyses that would increase the probability of making an incorrect decision while falsely assuming that each analysis is orthogonal. More variables also can be analyzed within a single multivariate test, thereby reducing the risk of Type I errors (rejecting the null hypothesis too easily), which can be thought of as liberal, assertive, and exploratory (Mulaik, Raju, & Harshman, 1997). We also can reduce Type II errors (retaining the null hypothesis too easily), which may be described as conservative, cautious, and confirmatory (Abelson, 1995). Analyzing more variables in a single analysis also minimizes the amount of unexplained or random error while maximizing the amount of explained systematic variance, which provides a much more realistic and rigorous framework for analyzing our data than with univariate methods.

e. *Fifth, multivariate thinking reveals several assessment indices to determine whether the overall or macro-analysis, as well as specific part or micro-analysis, are behaving as expected.* These overall and specific aspects encompass both omnibus (e.g., F-test) and specific (e.g., Tukey) tests of significance, along with associated effect sizes (e.g., eta-squared and Cohen's d). Acknowledging the wide debate of significance testing (Berkson, 1942;

Cohen, 1994; Harlow, Mulaik & Steiger, 1997; Kline, 2004; Meehl, 1978; Morrison & Henkel, 1970; Schmidt, 1996), I concur with recommendations for their tempered use along with supplemental information such as effect sizes (Abelson, 1997; Cohen, 1988, 1992; Kirk, 1996; Mulaik, Raju & Harshman, 1997; Thompson, 1996; Wilkinson & the APA Task Force on Statistical Inference, 1999). In Chapter 2 we discuss the topic of macro- and micro-assessment in greater detail to help interpret findings from multivariate analyses.

f. *Finally, multivariate participation in the research process engenders more positive attitudes toward statistics in general.* Active involvement increases our confidence in critiquing others' research and gives us more enthusiasm for applying methods to our own research. Greater feeling of empowerment occurs with less anticipatory anxiety when approaching statistics and research. We may well find ourselves asking more complex research questions with greater assurance, thereby increasing our own understanding. All this should help us to feel more comfortable articulating multiple ideas in an intelligent manner and to engage less in doubting our own capabilities with statistics and research. This is consequential because the bounty of multivariate information available could instill trepidation in many who would rather not delve into it without some coaxing. However, my experience has been that more exposure to the capabilities and applications of multivariate methods empowers us to pursue greater understanding and hopefully to provide greater contributions to the body of scientific knowledge.

DRAWBACKS

Because of the size and complexity of most multivariate designs, several drawbacks may be evident. I present three drawbacks that could emerge when thinking about multivariate methods and end with two additional drawbacks that are more tongue-in-cheek perceptions that could result:

a. *First, statistical assumptions (e.g., normality, linearity, and homoscedasticity) common to the general linear model (McCullagh & Nelder, 1989) must be met for most multivariate methods.* Less is known about the robustness of these to violations compared with univariate methods. More is said about assumptions in the section on Inferential Statistics in Chapter 3.

b. *Second, many more participants are usually needed to adequately test a multivariate design compared with smaller univariate studies.* One guideline suggests having 5 to 10 participants per variable or per parameter, although as many as 20 to 50 participants per variable or parameter may be necessary when assumptions are not met (Bentler, 1995; Tabachnick & Fidell, 2001). Others (Boomsma, 1983;

Comrey & Lee, 1992) recommend having a sample size of 200-500, with smaller sample sizes allowed when there are large effect sizes (Green, 1991; Guadagnoli & Velicer, 1988).

    c. *Third, interpretation of results from a multivariate analysis may be difficult because of having several layers to examine.* With multivariate methods, we can often examine:

      i. The overall significance to assess the probability that results were due to chance;

      ii. The main independent variables that are contributing to the analysis;

      iii. The nature of the dependent variable(s) showing significance; and

      iv. The specific pattern of the relationship between relevant independent and dependent variables.

    d. *Fourth, some researchers speculate that multivariate methods are too complex to take the time to learn.* That is an inaccurate perception because the basic themes are clear and reoccurring, as we will shortly see.

    e. *Fifth, after immersing ourselves in multivariate thinking, it could become increasingly difficult to justify constructing or analyzing a narrow and unrealistic research study.* We might even find ourselves thinking from a much wider and global perspective.

CONTEXT FOR MULTIVARIATE THINKING

The main focus of learning and education is knowledge consumption and development in which we are taught about the order that others have uncovered and learn methods to seek our own vision of order. During our early years, we are largely consumers of others' knowledge, learning from experts about what is important and how it can be understood. As we develop in our education, we move more into knowledge development and generation, which is explored and fine-tuned through the practice of scientific research. The learning curve for research can be very slow, although both interest and expertise increase with exposure and involvement. After a certain point, which widely varies depending on individual interests and instruction, the entire process of research clicks and becomes unbelievably compelling. We become hooked, getting a natural high from the process of discovery, creation, and verification of scientific knowledge. I personally believe all of us are latent scientists of sorts, if only at an informal level. We each go about making hypotheses about everyday events and situations, based on more or less formal theories. We then collect evidence for or against these hypotheses and make conclusions and future predictions based on our findings. When this process is formalized and validated in well-supported and well-structured environments, the opportunity for a major contribution by a well-informed individual becomes much more likely. Further, this is accompanied by a deeply felt sense of satisfaction and reward. That has certainly been my experience.

TABLE 1.1
Summary of the Definition, Benefits, Drawbacks, and Context for
Multivariate Methods

1. Definition	Set of tools for identifying relationships among multiple variables
2. Benefits	a. Stretch thinking to embrace a larger context
	b. Help in understanding others' research
	c. Expand capabilities with our own research
	d. Examine large sets of variables in a single analysis
	e. Provide several macro- and micro-assessment indices
	f. Engender more positive attitudes toward statistics in general
3. Drawbacks	a. Less is known about robustness of multivariate assumptions
	b. Larger sample sizes are needed
	c. Results are sometimes more complex to interpret
	d. Methods may be challenging to learn
	e. Broader focus requires more expansive thinking
4. Context	a. Knowledge consumption of others' research
	b. Knowledge generation from one's own research

Both knowledge-consuming and -generating endeavors, particularly in the social and behavioral sciences, are greatly enhanced by the study of multivariate thinking. One of our roles as multivariate social-behavioral scientists is to attempt to synthesize and integrate our understanding and knowledge in an area. Piecemeal strands of information are useful only to the extent that they eventually get combined to allow a larger, more interwoven fabric of comprehension to emerge. For example, isolated symptoms are of little value in helping an ailing patient unless a physician can integrate them into a well-reasoned diagnosis. Multivariate thinking helps us in this venture and allows us to clearly specify our understanding of a behavioral process or social phenomenon.

Table 1.1 summarizes the definition, benefits, drawbacks, and context for multivariate methods.

In the next chapter, we gain more specificity by taking note of various themes that run through all of multivariate thinking.

REFERENCES

Abelson, R. P. (1995). *Statistics as principled argument.* Mahwah, NJ: Lawrence Erlbaum Associates.
Abelson, R. P. (1997). The surprising longevity of flogged horses: Why there is a case for the significance test. *Psychological Science, 8,* 12–15.
Bentler, P. M. (1995). *EQS: Structural equations program manual.* Encino, CA: Multivariate Software, Inc.
Berkson, J. (1942). Tests of significance considered as evidence. *Journal of the American Statistical Association, 37,* 325–335.
Boomsma, A. (1983). *On the robustness of LISREL (maximum likelihood estimation) against small sample size and nonnormality.* PhD. Thesis, University of Groningen, The Netherlands.

Cohen, J. (1988). *Statistical power analysis for the behavioral sciences*. San Diego, CA: Academic Press.

Cohen, J. (1992). A power primer. *Psychological Bulletin, 112*, 155-159.

Cohen, J. (1994). The earth is round (p < .05). *American Psychologist, 49*, 997–1003.

Cohen, J., Cohen, P., West, S. G., & Aiken, L. S. (2003). *Applied multiple regression/correlation analysis for behavioral sciences* (3rd ed.). Mahwah, NJ: Lawrence Erlbaum Associates.

Comrey, A. L., & Lee, H. B. (1992). *A first course in factor analysis* (2nd ed.). Hillsdale, NJ: Lawrence Erlbaum Associates.

Gorsuch, R. L. (1999). *UniMult: For univariate and multivariate data analysis (Computer program and guide)*. Pasadena, CA: UniMult.

Green, S. B. (1991). How many subjects does it take to do a regression analysis? *Multivariate Behavioral Research, 26*, 449–510.

Guadagnoli, E., & Velicer, W. F. (1988). Relation of sample size to the stability of component patterns. *Psychological Bulletin, 10*, 265–275.

Harlow, L. L., Mulaik S. A., & Steiger, J. H. (1997). *What if there were no significance tests?* Mahwah, NJ: Lawrence Erlbaum Associates.

Harris, R. J. (2001). *A primer of multivariate statistics*. Mahwah, NJ: Lawrence Erlbaum Associates.

Kirk, R. E. (1996). Practical significance: A concept whose time has come. *Educational and Psychological Measurement, 56*, 746–759.

Kline, R. B. (2004). *Beyond significance testing: Reforming data analysis methods in behavioral research*. Washington DC: APA.

Marcoulides, G. A., & Hershberger, S. L. (1997). *Multivariate statistical methods: A first course*. Mahwah, NJ: Lawrence Erlbaum Associates.

McCullagh, P., & Nelder, J. (1989). *Generalized linear models*. London: Chapman and Hall.

Meehl, P. E. (1978). Theoretical risks and tabular asterisks: Sir Karl, Sir Ronald, and the slow progress of soft psychology. *Journal of Consulting and Clinical Psychology, 46*, 806–834.

Morrison, D. E., & Henkel, R. E. (Eds.) (1970). *The significance test controversy*. Chicago: Aldine.

Mulaik, S. A., Raju, N. S., & Harshman, R. A. (1997). A time and place for significance testing. In L. L. Harlow, S. A. Mulaik, & J. H. Steiger (Eds.), *What if there were no significance tests?* (pp. 65–115). Mahwah, NJ: Lawrence Erlbaum Associates.

Schmidt, F. L. (1996). Statistical significance testing and cumulative knowledge in psychology: Implications for the training of researchers. *Psychological Methods, 1*, 115–129.

Simon, H. A. (1969). *The sciences of the artificial*. Cambridge, MA: The M.I.T. Press.

Tabachnick, B. G., & Fidell, L. S. (2001). *Using multivariate statistics* (4th ed.). Boston: Allyn and Bacon.

Thompson, B. (1996). AERA editorial policies regarding statistical significance testing: Three suggested reforms. *Educational Researcher, 25*, 26–30.

Wheatley, M. J. (1994). *Leadership and the new science: Learning about organization from an orderly universe*. San Francisco, DA: Berrett-Koehler Publishers, Inc.

Wilkinson, L., & the APA Task Force on Statistical Inference (1999). Statistical methods in psychology journals: Guidelines and explanations. *American Psychologist, 54*, 594–604.

2

Multivariate Themes

Quantitative methods have long been heralded for their ability to synthesize the basic meaning in a body of knowledge. Aristotle emphasized meaning through the notion of "definition" as the set of necessary and sufficient properties that allowed an unfolding of understanding about concrete or abstract phenomena; Plato thought of essence or meaning as the basic form (Lakoff & Núñez, 2000). Providing insight into central meaning is at the heart of most mathematics, which uses axioms and categorical forms to define the nature of specific mathematical systems.

This chapter focuses on the delineation of basic themes that reoccur within statistics, particularly with multivariate procedures, in the hope of making conscious and apprehensible the core tenets, if not axioms, of multivariate thinking.

OVERRIDING THEME OF MULTIPLICITY

The main theme of multivariate thinking is multiplicity, drawing on multiple sources in the development of a strong methodology. We are ultimately looking for truth in multiple places and in multiple ways. We could start by identifying multiple ways of thinking about a system; for example, we could consider how theory, empirical research, and applied practice impinge on our study. If there is a strong, theoretical framework that guides our research, rigorous empirical methods with which to test our hypotheses, and practical implications that derive from our findings, contributions to greater knowledge and understanding become much more likely. We also could investigate multiple ways to measure our constructs, multiple statistical methods to test our hypotheses, multiple controls to ensure clear conclusions, and multiple time points and samples with which to generalize our results. We might argue that the extent to which a research study incorporated the concept of multiplicity, the more rigorous, generalizable, reliable, and valid the results would be.

In our multivariate venture into knowledge generation within the social sciences, perhaps the most primary goal is to consider several relevant theories that could direct our efforts to understand a phenomenon.

Theory

Before embarking on a research study, it is essential to inquire about meta-frameworks that can provide a structure with which to conduct our research. Are there multiple divergent perspectives to consider? Are any of them more central or salient than the others? Which seem to offer a more encompassing way to view an area of study while also providing a basis for strong investigations? Meehl (1997) talks of the need to draw on theory that makes risky predictions that are capable of being highly refuted. These strong theories are much preferred to weak ones that make vague and vacuous propositions. Others concur with Meehl's emphasis on theory. Wilson (1998) speaks of theory in reverent words, stating that "Nothing in science—nothing in life, for that matter—makes sense without theory. It is our nature to put all knowledge into context in order to tell a story, and to re-create the world by this means" (p. 56). Theory provides a coherent theme to help us find meaning and purpose in our research. Wheatley (1994) speaks of the power and coherence of theory in terms of providing an overall meaning and focus in our research. She writes, "As long as we keep purpose in focus . . . we are able to wander through the realms of chaos . . . and emerge with a discernible pattern or shape." (p. 136). Abelson (1995) discusses theory as being able to cull together a wide range of findings into "coherent bundles of results" (p. 14). Thus, a thorough understanding of the theories that are germane to our research will provide purpose and direction in our quest to perceive the pattern of meaning that is present in a set of relevant variables. This level of theoretical understanding makes it more likely that meaningful hypotheses can be posited that are grounded in a coherent structure and framework.

Hypotheses

Upon pondering a number of theories of a specific phenomenon, several hypotheses or predictions undoubtedly will emerge. In our everyday life, we all formulate predictions and hypotheses, however informal. This can be as mundane as a prediction about what will happen during our day or how the weather will unfold. In scientific research, we strive to formalize our hypotheses so that they directly follow from well-thought-out theory. The more specific and precise our hypotheses, the more likelihood there is of either refuting them or finding useful evidence to corroborate them (Meehl, 1997). Edward O. Wilson (1998) makes this clear by stating that theoretical tests of hypotheses "are constructed specifically to be blown apart if proved wrong, and if so destined, the sooner the better" (p. 57). Multivariate statistics allows us to formulate multiple hypotheses that can be tested in conjunction. Thus, we should try to formulate several pivotal hypotheses or research questions that allow for rigorous tests of our theories, allowing us to hone and fine-tune our theories or banish them as useless (Wilson, 1998). The testing of these hypotheses is the work of empirical research.

Empirical Studies

Having searched out pertinent theories that lead to strong predictions, it is important to investigate what other researchers have found in our area of research. Are there multiple empirical studies that have previously touched on aspects of these theories and predictions? Are there multiple contributions that could be made with new research that would add to the empirical base in this area? Schmidt and Hunter (1997) emphasize the need to accrue results from multiple studies and assess them within a meta-analysis framework. This allows the regularities and consistent ideas to emerge as a larger truth than could be found from single studies. Abelson (1995) describes this as the development of "the lore" whereby "well-articulated research . . . is likely to be absorbed and repeated by other investigators" as a collective understanding of a phenomenon (pp. 105–106). No matter what the empirical area of interest, a thorough search of previous research on a topic should illuminate the core constructs that could be viewed as pure or meta-versions of our specific variables of interest. After taking into account meaningful theories, hypotheses, and empirical studies we are ready to consider how to measure the major constructs we plan to include in our research.

Measurement

When conducting empirical research, it is useful to ask about the nature of measurement for constructs of interest (McDonald, 1999; Pedhazur & Schmelkin, 1991). Are there several pivotal constructs that need to be delineated and measured? Are there multiple ways to measure each of these constructs? Are there multiple, different items or variables for each of these measures? *Classical test theory* (Lord & Novick, 1968) and *item response theory* (Embretson, & Reise, 2000; McDonald, 2000) emphasize the importance of modeling the nature of an individual's response to a measure and the properties of the measures. *Reliability theory* (Anastasi & Urbina, 1997; Lord & Novick, 1968; McDonald, 1999) emphasizes the need to have multiple items for each scale or subscale we wish to measure. Similarly, statistical analysts conducting principal components or factor analyses emphasize the need for a minimum of three or four variables to anchor each underlying dimension or construct (Gorsuch, 1983; Velicer & Jackson, 1990). The more variables we use, the more likelihood there is that we are tapping the true dimension of interest. In everyday terms, this is comparable to realizing that we cannot expect someone else to know who we are if we use only one or two terms to describe ourselves. Certainly, students would agree that if a teacher were to ask just a single exam question to tap all their knowledge in a topic area, this would hardly begin to do the trick. Multivariate thinking aids us in this regard by not only encouraging but also requiring multiple variables to be examined in conjunction. This makes it much more likely that we will come to a deeper understanding of the phenomenon under study. Having identified several pertinent variables, it also is important to consider whether there are multiple time points across which a set of variables can be analyzed.

Multiple Time Points

Does a phenomenon change over time? Does a certain period of time need to pass before a pattern emerges or takes form? These questions often are important when we want to examine change or stability over time (Collins, & Horn, 1991; Collins, & Sayer, 2001; Moskowitz, & Hershberger, 2002). Assessing samples at multiple time points aids us in discerning which variables are most likely the causal agents and which are the receptive outcomes. If the magnitude of a relationship is always stronger when one variable precedes another in time, there is some evidence that the preceding (i.e., independent) variable may be affecting the other, more dependent outcome. Having contemplated the possibility of multiple time points, it is important to consider how to build in multiple controls.

Multiple Controls

Perhaps the best way to ensure causal inferences is to implement controls within a research design (Pearl, 2000). The three most salient controls involve a test of clear association between variables, evidence of temporal ordering of the variables, and the ability to rule out potential confounds or extraneous variables (Bullock, Harlow, & Mulaik, 1994). This can be achieved most elegantly with an experimental design that:

1. Examines the association between carefully selected reliable variables,
2. Manipulates the independent variable so that one or more groups receive a treatment, whereas at least one group does not, and
3. Randomly selects a sufficient number of participants from a relevant population and randomly assigns them to either the treatment or the control group.

With this kind of design, there is a greater likelihood that nonspurious relationships will emerge in which the independent variable can definitively be identified as the causal factor, with potential confounding variables safely ruled out with the random selection and assignment (Fisher, 1925, 1926).

Despite the virtues of an experimental design in ensuring control over one's research, it is often difficult to enact such a design. Variables, particularly those used in social sciences, cannot always be easily manipulated. For example, I would loathe to experimentally manipulate the amount of substance abuse that is needed to bring about a sense of meaninglessness in life. These kinds of variables would be examined more ethically in a quasi-experimental design that tried to systematically rule out relevant confounds (Shadish, Cook, & Campbell, 2002). These types of designs could include background variables (e.g., income, education, age at first substance abuse, history of substance abuse, history of meaninglessness), or covariates (e.g., network of substance users in one's environment, stressful life events) that could be statistically controlled while examining the relationship perceived between independent variables (IVs) and dependent variables (DVs). Needless to say, it is very difficult to ensure that adequate controls are in place without an experimental design, although the realities of real-world research make it necessary to consider alternative designs. In addition to multiple controls, it is useful to consider collecting data from multiple samples.

Multiple Samples

Are there several pertinent populations or samples from which data could be gathered to empirically study the main constructs and hypotheses? Samples are a subset of entities (e.g., persons) from which we obtain data to statistically analyze. Ideally, samples are drawn randomly from a relevant population, although much research is conducted with convenience samples, such as classrooms of students. Another type of sampling is called "purposive," which refers to forming a sample that is purposely heterogeneous or typical of the kind of population from which generalization is possible (Shadish, Cook & Campbell, 2002). When samples are not drawn at random or purposively, it is difficult to generalize past the sample to a larger population (Shadish, 1995). Still, results from a nonrandom sample can offer descriptive or preliminary information that can be followed up in other research. Procedures such as propensity score analysis (Rosenbaum, 2002) can be used to identify covariates that can address selection bias in a nonrandom sample, thus allowing the possibility of generalizing to a larger population. The importance of identifying relevant and meaningful samples is pivotal to all research. Further, in multivariate research, samples are usually larger than when fewer variables are examined.

Whether analyzing univariate or multivariate data from a relevant sample, it is preferable to verify whether the findings are consistent. Fisher (1935) highlighted the need for replicating findings in independent samples. Further, researchers (Collyer, 1986; Cudeck & Browne, 1983) reiterate the importance of demonstrating that findings can be cross-validated. Statistical procedures have been developed in several areas of statistics that incorporate findings from multiple samples. For example, Jöreskog (1971) and Sörbom (1974) developed multiple sample procedures for assessing whether a hypothesized mathematical model holds equally well in more than one sample. These multiple sample procedures allow for tests of increasing rigor of replication or equality across the samples, starting with a test of an equal pattern of relationships among hypothesized constructs, up through equality of sets of parameters (e.g., factor loadings, regressions, and means) among constructs. If a hypothesized model can be shown to hold equally well across multiple samples, particularly when constraining the parameters to be the same, this provides a strong test of the generalizability of a model (Alwin & Jackson, 1981; Bentler, Lee & Weng, 1987; Jöreskog, 1971). Even if many multivariate methods do not have specific procedures for cross-validating findings, efforts should be taken to ensure that results would generalize to multiple samples, thus allowing greater confidence in their applicability.

Practical Implications

Although research does not have to fill an immediately apparent practical need, it is helpful to consider what implications can be derived from a body of research. When multiple variables are examined, there is a greater likelihood that connections among them will manifest in ways that suggest practical applications. For example, research in health sciences often investigates multiple plausible predictors of disease, or conversely well-being (Diener & Suh, 2000), that can be used in developing interventions to prevent illness and sustain positive health (Prochaska & Velicer, 1997; Velicer et al., 2000). Practical applications do not have to originate with initial research in an area. For example, John Nash researched mathematical group theory, which only later was used to understand economics, bringing Nash a Nobel Prize (Nash, 2002). Lastly, it is important to consider a number of multivariate methods from which we can select for specific research goals.

Multiple Statistical Methods

Are several analyses needed to address the main questions? What kinds of analyses are needed? It is often important to examine research by using several multivariate methods (Grimm & Yarnold, 1995, 2000; Marcoulides & Hershberger, 1997; Tabachnick & Fidell, 2001). John Tukey (1977) championed the idea of liberally exploring our data to find what it could reveal to us. In this respect, it is not unlike an artist using several tools and utensils to work with a mound of clay until the underlying form and structure is made manifest. Throughout the book, examples are provided about how the themes pertain to various multivariate methods. Here, a brief overview of several kinds of multivariate methods is given.

One set of methods focuses on group differences (Maxwell & Delaney, 2004; Tabachnick & Fidell, 2001). For all these group difference methods, the main question is Are there mean significant differences across groups over and above what would occur by random chance, and how much of a relationship is there between the grouping and outcome variables? Analysis of covariance (ANCOVA) allows examination of group differences on a single outcome after controlling for the effects of one or more continuous covariates. Multivariate analysis of variance

(MANOVA) is used to examine group differences on linear combinations of several continuous DVs. Each of these group difference methods help us discern whether the average score between each group is more different than the scores within each group. If the between-group differences are greater than the random differences found among scores within each group, we have some evidence that the nature of the group is associated with the outcome scores. This is useful information, especially when resources are scarce or decisions need to be made that affect specific groups. For example, it is important to be able to differentiate groups that do and do not need medical treatment, educational enrichment, or psychological interventions.

Prediction methods allow us to predict an outcome on the basis of several predictor variables. The main question addressed with these methods is How much of an outcome can we know given a set of predictor variables, and is the degree of relationship significantly different from zero?

When there are a set of predictors and a single continuous outcome variable, multiple regression (MR) (Cohen, Cohen, West, & Aiken, 2003) is the method of choice. If there are multiple predictors and a categorical outcome and assumptions of normality (i.e., bell-shaped multivariate distribution) and homoscedasticity (i.e., equal variances on one variable at each level of another variable) hold, discriminant function analysis (DFA) (Tatsuoka, 1970) can be used. With a mix of categorical and continuous predictors that do not necessarily adhere to statistical assumptions, logistic regression (LR) (Hosmer & Lemeshow, 2000) offers another way to ascertain the probability of a categorical outcome. When there are multiple predictors and outcomes, canonical correlation (CC) may be useful to explore the degree of relationship between the two sets of variables. Each of these predictive methods allows us to assess possible relationships between variables, so that scores increase or decrease in predictable ways. If the pattern of increase and decrease between two sets of scores is almost as large as the average random differences among the scores for each variable, there is some evidence of an association between the pair(s) of variables. Prediction methods are helpful in determining which set of variables is most closely linked to a specific outcome. For example, it would be useful to predict who will do well in recovering from a disease or in achieving success in an educational or business environment.

Exploratory dimensional methods delineate the underlying dimensions in a large set of variables or individuals. When the goal is to reduce a large set of correlated variables to a smaller set of orthogonal dimensions then principal components analysis (PCA) is appropriate (Velicer & Jackson, 1990). When the focus is on identifying a set of theoretical dimensions that explain the shared common variance in a set of variables, factor analysis (FA) can be used (Gorsuch, 1983; McDonald, 1985). These analyses can help delineate the main dimensions that underlie a large set of variables. For example, we could identify several dimensions to explain a large number of items measuring various facets of intelligence by using PCA or FA.

TABLE 2.1
Summary of Multivariate Themes

1. Multiplicity Themes (Multiple considerations at all levels of focus, with greater multiplicity generally leading to greater reliability, validity, and generalization)	a. Multiple theories b. Multiple empirical studies c. Multiple hypotheses d. Multiple measures e. Multiple time points f. Multiple controls g. Multiple samples h. Practical implications i. Multiple statistical methods
2. Central Themes (All multivariate methods focus on these central themes)	a. Variance b. Covariance c. Ratios of variance (and covariance) d. Linear combinations (e.g., components, factors)
3. Interpretation Themes (Big picture and specific levels)	a. Macro-assessment (e.g., significance test and effect size) b. Micro-assessment (e.g., examining means or weights)

Summary of Multiplicity Themes

In the realm of methodology, each of these facets of multiplicity (see Table 2.1) coalesce or come together under the effective tools of multivariate statistics to inform us of the fundamental nature of the phenomenon under study. All considered investigation begins with well-reasoned theories, articulate hypotheses, careful empirical research, accurate measurement, representative samples, and relevant statistical methods. When time and multiple controls are possible, we also may be able to discern the causal nature of the relationships among variables.

CENTRAL THEMES

Just as with basic descriptive and inferential statistics, multivariate methods help us understand and quantify how variables (co-)vary. Multivariate methods provide a set of tools to analyze how scores from several variables covary—whether through group differences, correlations, or underlying dimensions—to explain systematic variance over and above random error variance. Thus, we are trying to explain or make sense of the variance in a set of variables with as little random error variance as possible. Multivariate methods draw on the multiplicity theme just discussed, with several additional themes. Probably the most central themes, for either multivariate or univariate methods, involve the concepts of variance, covariance, and ratios of these (co-)variances. We also will examine the theme of creating linear combinations of the variables, because this is central to most multivariate methods.

Variance

Variance is the average of the squared difference between a set of scores and their mean. Variance is what we usually want to analyze with any statistic. When a variable has a large variance, sample scores tend to be very different, having a wide range. It is useful to try to predict how scores vary, to find other variables that help explain the variation. Statistical methods help identify systematic, explained variance, acknowledging that there most likely will be a portion of unknowable and random (e.g., error) variance. The goal of most statistics is to try to explain how scores vary so that we can predict or understand them better. Variance is an important theme, particularly in multivariate thinking, and it can be analyzed in several ways, as we shall see later in this chapter.

Covariance

Covariance is the product of the average differences between one variable and its mean and a second variable and its mean. Covariance or its standardized form, correlation, depicts the existence of a linear relationship between two or more variables. When variables rise and fall together (e.g., study time and grade point average), they positively covary or co-relate. If scores vary in opposite directions (e.g., greater practice is associated with a lower golf score), negative covariance occurs. The theme of covariation is fundamental to multivariate methods, because we are interested in whether a set of variables tend to co-occur together, indicating a strong relationship. Multivariate methods most often assess covariance by assessing the relationship among variables while also taking into account the covariation among other variables included in the analysis. Thus, multivariate methods allow a more informed test of the relationships among variables than can be analyzed with univariate methods that expect separate or orthogonal relationships with other variables.

Ratio of (Co-)Variances

Many methods examine a ratio of how much (co-)variance there is between variables or groups relative to how much variance there is within variables or within groups. When the between information is large relative to the within information, we usually conclude that the results are significantly different from those that could be found based on pure chance. The reason for this is that when there are greater differences across domains than there are within domains, whether from different variables or different groups, there is some indication of systematic shared or associated variance that is not just attributable to random error.

It is useful to see how correlation and ANOVA, two central, univariate statistical methods, embody a ratio of variances. We can then extend this thinking to multivariate methods. Correlation shows a ratio of covariance between variables over variance within variables. When the covariance between variables is almost as large as the variance within either variable, this indicates a stronger relationship between variables. Thus, a large correlation indicates that much of the variance within each variable is shared or covaries between the variables.

With group difference statistics (e.g., ANOVA), we often form an F-ratio of how much the group means vary relative to how much variance there is within each group. When the means are much more different between groups (i.e., large variance between groups) than the scores are within each group (i.e., smaller variance within groups), we have evidence of a relationship between the grouping (e.g., categorical, independent) and outcome (e.g., continuous, dependent) variables. Here, a large F-ratio indicates significant group difference variance.

These ratios, whether correlational or ANOVA-based, are also found in multivariate methods. In fact, just about every statistical significance test is based on some kind of ratio of variances or covariances. Knowing this fact and understanding the nature of the ratio for each analysis helps us make much more sense out of our statistical results, whether from univariate or multivariate methods.

Linear Combinations

A basic theme throughout most multivariate methods is that of finding the relationship between two or more sets of variables. This usually is accomplished by forming linear combinations of the variables in each set that are additive composites that maximize the amount of variance drawn from the variables. A simple example of a linear combination is the course grade received in many classes. The grade, let's call it X', is formed from the weighted combination of various scores. Thus, a course grading scheme of $X' = 0.25$ (homework) $+ 0.25$ (midterm exam) $+ 0.30$ (final exam) $+ 0.20$ (project) would reveal a linear combination showing the weights attached to the four course requirements.

These linear combination scores are then analyzed, summarizing the many variables in a simple, concise form. With multivariate methods, we often are trying to assess the relationship between variables, which is often the shared variance between linear combinations of variables. Several multivariate methods analyze different kinds of linear combinations.

Components

A component is a linear combination of variables that maximizes the variance extracted from the original set of variables. The concept of forming linear combinations is most salient with PCA (see Chapter 11 for more on PCA). With PCA, we aim to find several linear combinations (i.e., components) that help explain most of the variance in a set of the original variables. MANOVA and DFA (see

Chapters 7 and 8, respectively) also form component-like linear combinations (i.e., discriminant scores) to examine the relationships among the categorical grouping variable(s) and the continuous, measured variables. CC (see Chapter 10) also forms linear combination components (i.e., canonical variates) for the predictors and for the outcomes, relating these to variables and other combinations within and across the two sets of continuous variables. MR (see Chapter 4) could be thought of as a subset of CC in which there is just a single linear combination or component. In each case, the use of components or linear combinations helps to synthesize information by redistributing most of the variance from a larger set of variables, usually into a smaller set of summary scores.

Factors

We have just seen how linear combinations can be thought of as dimensions that seem to summarize the essence of a set of variables. If we are conducting a FA, we refer to these dimensions as factors. Factors differ from the linear combinations analyzed in PCA, MANOVA, DFA, and CC in that they are more latent dimensions that have separated common, shared variance among the variables from any unique or measurement error variance within the variables. Thus, a factor sometimes is believed to represent the underlying true dimension in a set of variables, after removing the portion of variance in the variables that is not common to the others (i.e., the unique or error portion). Exploratory FA is discussed in the current text, (see Chapter 10) although there are confirmatory FA procedures that are also relevant and will be left for another volume.

Summary of Central Themes

In the discussion of central themes, we saw the pivotal role of variances, covariances and ratios of these, particularly in multivariate statistics. Ultimately, we are always trying to explain how variables vary and covary, and we do so often by examining a ratio of variances or covariances. The ratio informs us of the proportion of explained variance that is often used as an indication of effect size. We also considered the concept of a linear combination that incorporates much of the variance from several variables. Several multivariate methods (e.g., PCA, FA, DFA, MANOVA, CC) use linear combinations to summarize information in sets of variables. Depending on the method, linear combinations are referred to with different terms (e.g., components, factors, discriminant functions, and canonical variates). Regardless of the label, multivariate linear combinations synthesize the information in a larger set of variables to make analyses more manageable or comprehensible. Now we turn to ways to evaluate and interpret results from multivariate methods, using both a macro- and micro-assessment focus.

INTERPRETATION THEMES

When interpreting results and assessing whether an analysis is successful, we should evaluate from several perspectives. Most statistical procedures, whether we are using univariate or multivariate methods, allow a macro-assessment of how well the overall analysis explains the variance among pertinent variables. It is also important to focus on a micro-assessment of the specific aspects of the multivariate results.

In keeping with ongoing debates about problems with the exclusive use of significance testing (Harlow, Mulaik, & Steiger, 1997; Kline, 2004; Wilkinson, & the APA Task Force on Statistical Inference, 1999), I advocate that each result be evaluated with both a significance test and an effect size whenever possible; that is, it is helpful to know whether a finding is significantly different from chance and to know the magnitude of the significant effect.

Macro-Assessment

The first way to evaluate an analysis is at a global or macro-level that usually involves a significance test and most likely some synthesis of the variance in a multivariate dataset. A *macro summary* usually depicts whether there is significant covariation or mean differences within data, relative to how much variation there is among scores within specific groups or variables.

Significance Test

A significance test, along with an accompanying probability or *p* value is usually the first step of macro-assessment in a multivariate design (Wilkinson, & the APA Task Force on Statistical Inference, 1999). Significance tests tell us whether our empirical results are likely to be due to random chance or not. It is useful to be able to rule out, with some degree of certainty, an accidental or anomalous finding. Of course, we always risk making an error no matter what our decision. When we accept our finding too easily, we could be guilty of a Type I error, saying that our research had veracity when in fact it was a random finding. When we are too cautious about accepting our findings, we may be committing a Type II error, saying that we have no significant findings when in fact we do. Significance tests help us to make probabilistic decisions about our results within an acceptable margin of error, usually set at 1% to 5%. We would like to say that we have more reason to believe our results are true than that they are not true. Significance tests give us some assurance in this regard, and they are essential when we have imperfect knowledge or a lack of certainty about an area. We can help rule out false starts and begin to accrue a growing knowledge base with these tests (Mulaik, Raju & Harshman, 1997).

Most univariate and multivariate significance tests imply a ratio of (co-)variances. For example, group difference methods (e.g., ANOVA, ANCOVA, MANOVA, MANCOVA, DFA) tend to use an F-test, which is a ratio of the variance between means over the variance within scores, to assess whether observed differences are significantly different from what we would expect based on chance alone. Correlational methods (e.g., MR, CC) also can make use of an F-test to assess whether the covariance among variables is large relative to the variance within variables. When the value of an F-test is significantly large (as determined by consulting appropriate statistical tables), we can conclude that there is sufficient evidence of relationships occurring at the macro-level. This suggests there is a goodness of approximation between the model and the data (McDonald, 1997). When this occurs, it is helpful to quantify the extent of the relationship, usually with effect sizes.

Effect Sizes

Effect sizes provide an indication of the magnitude of our findings at an overall level. They are a useful supplement to the results of a significance test (Wilkinson & the APA Task Force on Statistical Inference, 1999). Effect size (ES) calculations can be standardized differences between means for group difference questions (e.g., Cohen's d) (Cohen, 1992; Kirk, 1996). Guidelines for interpreting small, medium, and large ESs are Cohen's d values of 0.2, 0.5, and 0.8, respectively (Cohen, 1988). Quite often, an ES takes the form of a proportion of shared variance between the independent and the dependent variables, particularly for multivariate analyses. Guidelines for multivariate shared variance are 0.02, 0.13, and 0.26 for small, medium, and large ESs, respectively (Cohen, 1992). Although much more can be said about effect sizes (Cohen, 1988), we focus largely on those that involve a measure of shared variance.

Shared variance is a common theme throughout most statistical methods and often can form the basis of an ES. We are always trying to understand how to explain the extent by which scores vary or covary. Almost always, this involves two sets of variables so that the focus is on how much variance is shared between the two sets (e.g., a set of IVs and a set of DVs, or a set of components-factors and a set of measured variables). With multivariate methods, one of the main ways of summarizing the essence of shared variance is with squared multiple correlations. Indices of shared variance or squared multiple correlations can inform us of the strength of relationship or effect size (Cohen, 1988).

Squared multiple correlation, R^2, indicates the amount of shared variance between the variables. It is useful by providing a single number that conveys how much the scores from a set of variables (co-)vary in the same way (i.e., rise and fall together) relative to how much the scores within each variable differ among themselves. A large R^2 value (e.g., 0.26 or greater) indicates that the participants' responses on a multivariate set of variables tend to behave similarly, so that a common or shared phenomenon may be occurring among the variables. For example, research by Richard and Shirley Jessor (1973) and their colleagues have demonstrated large proportions of shared variance between alcohol abuse, drug abuse, risky sexual behavior, and psychosocial variables, providing compelling evidence that an underlying phenomenon of "problem behavior" is apparent.

Many statistical methods make use of the concept of R^2 or shared variance. Pearson's correlation coefficient, r, is an index of the strength of relationship between two variables. Squaring this correlation yields R^2, sometimes referred to as a coefficient of determination that indicates how much overlapping variance is shared between two variables. In MR (Cohen, Cohen, West, & Aiken, 2003), a powerful multivariate method useful for prediction, we can use R^2 to examine how much variance is shared between a linear combination of several independent variables and a single outcome variable. The linear combination for MR (see Chapter 4) is formed by a least-squares approach that minimizes the squared difference between actual and predicted outcome scores. In Chapter 6, we will see how shared variance across linear combinations can be summarized with functions of eigenvalues, traces, or determinants, each of which is described in the discussion of matrix notation and calculations.

Residual or error variance is another possible consideration when discussing central themes. Many statistical procedures benefit from assessing the amount of residual or error variance in an analysis. In prediction methods, such as MR (see Chapter 4), we often want to examine prediction error variance (i.e., $1 - R^2$), which is how much variation in the outcome variable was not explained by the predictors. In MANOVA, DFA, and CC (see Chapters 7, 8 and 10), we can approximate the residuals by subtracting eta squared (i.e., η^2: ratio of between variance to total variance) from one, also known as Wilks's (1932) lambda.

Micro-Assessment

After finding significant results and a meaningful ES at a macro-level, it is then useful to examine results at a more specific, micro-level. Micro-assessment involves examining specific facets of an analysis (e.g., means, weights) to determine specifically what is contributing to the overall relationship. In micro-assessment, we ask whether there are specific coefficients or values that can shed light on which aspects of the system are working and which are not.

Means

With group difference methods, micro-assessment entails an examination of the differences between pairs of means. We can accomplish this by simply presenting a descriptive summary of the means and standard deviations for the variables across groups and possibly graphing them to allow visual examination of any trends. Several other methods are suggested for more formally assessing means.

1. **Standardized effect size for means.** Cohen's d (1988) is a useful micro-level ES, formed from the ratio of the difference between means divided by the (pooled) standard deviation. With the values given earlier (see *Effect Sizes*, above) (Cohen, 1988), a small ES indicates a mean difference of almost a quarter (i.e., 0.2) of a standard deviation. A medium ES is a mean difference of a half (i.e., 0.5) of a standard deviation. A large ES suggests almost a whole (i.e., 0.8) standard deviation difference between means.
2. **Bonferroni comparisons.** Simply conducting a series of t-tests between pairs of groups allows us to evaluate the significance of group means. A Bonferroni approach establishes a set alpha level (e.g., $p = 0.05$) and then distributes the available alpha level over the number of paired comparisons. Thus, if there were four comparisons and a desired alpha level of 0.05, each comparison of means could be equally evaluated with a p value of 0.0125. Of course the p value can be unevenly split (e.g., 0.02 for one comparison and 0.01 for three comparisons between means).
3. **Planned comparisons.** We could also see which pairs of means were statistically different by using a multiple comparison method such as Tukey's (1953) honestly significant difference approach that builds in control of Type I error. Ideally, these micro-level tests should directly follow from our hypotheses, rather than simply testing for any possible difference.
4. **Fisher's protected tests.** The practice of conducting an overall significance test and then following up with individual t-tests for pairs of means is referred to as a Fisher protected t-test (Carmer & Swanson, 1973). Whereas Bonferroni and planned comparison approaches are conservative and may not provide enough power to detect a meaningful effect, Fisher's protected approach often is preferred because of its ability to control experiment-wise Type I error and still find individual differences between pairs of means (Cohen, Cohen, West & Aiken, 2003).

Weights

With correlational or dimensional methods, we often want to examine weights that indicate how much of a specific variable is contributing to an analysis. In MR, we examine least-squares regression weights that tell us how much a predictor variable covaries with an outcome variable after taking into account the relationships with other predictor variables. In an unstandardized metric, it represents the change in an outcome variable that can be expected when a predictor variable is changed by one unit. In a standardized metric, the regression weight, often referred to as a beta weight, gives the partial correlation between the predictor and the outcome, after controlling for the other predictor variables in the equation. Thus, the weight provides an indication of the unique importance of a predictor with an outcome variable. In other multivariate methods (e.g., see DFA, CC, PCA in Chapters 8, 10, and 11), the unstandardized weights are actually eigenvector weights (see Chapter 6 on matrix notation) used in forming linear combinations of the variables. These are often standardized to provide an interpretation similar to the standardized weight in MR. In FA, weights are also examined. These can indicate the amount of relationship (i.e., a factor loading) between a variable and an underlying dimension. In each of these instances, the weight informs us how much a specific variable relates to some aspect of the analysis. The weight or the squared value of a weight also can be used as a micro-level ES for correlational methods. Guidelines for interpreting small, medium, and large micro-level shared variance ESs are 0.01, 0.06, and 0.13, respectively (Cohen, 1992).

Summary of Interpretation Themes

For most multivariate methods, there are two themes that help us with interpreting our results. The first of these, macro-assessment, focuses on whether the overall analysis is significant and on the magnitude of the effect size. In addition, we often want to examine residuals to assess the unexplained or error variance. The magnitude and nature of error variance informs us as to where and how much the multivariate method is not explaining the data. Second, micro-assessment focuses on the specific aspects of an analysis that are important in explaining the overall relationship. These micro-aspects can be means, particularly with group difference methods, or weights, particularly with correlational methods.

Summary of Multivariate Themes

In this chapter, several sets of themes were discussed to help in understanding the nature of multivariate methods. A summary of these themes is presented in Table 2.1.

REFERENCES

Abelson, R. P. (1995). *Statistics as principled argument.* Mahwah, NJ: Lawrence Erlbaum Associates.

Alwin, D. F., & Jackson, D. J. (1981). Applications of simultaneous factor analysis to issues of factorial invariance. In D. Jackson & E. Borgatta (Eds.), *Factor analysis and measurement in sociological research: A multi-dimensional perspective.* Beverly Hills: Sage Publications.

Anastasi, A., & Urbina, S. (1997). *Psychological testing.* Upper Saddle River, NJ: Prentice Hall.

Bentler, P. M., Lee, S.-Y., & Weng, L.-J. (1987). Multiple population covariance structure analysis under arbitrary distribution theory. *Communications in Statistics—Theory, 16,* 1951–1964.

Bullock, H. E., Harlow, L. L., & Mulaik, S. (1994). Causation issues in structural modeling research. *Structural Equation Modeling Journal, 1,* 253–267.

Carmer, S. G., & Swanson, M. R. (1973). An evaluation of ten pairwise multiple comparison procedures by Monte Carlo methods. *Journal of the American Statistical Association, 68,* 66–74.

Cohen, J. (1988). *Statistical power analysis for the behavioral sciences.* San Diego, CA: Academic Press.

Cohen, J. (1992). A power primer. *Psychological Bulletin, 112,* 155–159.

Cohen, J., Cohen, P., West, S. G., & Aiken, L. S. (2003). *Applied multiple regression/correlation analysis for behavioral sciences* (3rd ed.). Mahwah, NJ: Lawrence Erlbaum Associates.

Collins, L., & Horn, J. (Eds.) (1991). *Best methods for the analysis of change.* Washington, DC: APA Publications.

Collins, L. M., & Sayer, A. G. (Ed). (2001). *New methods for the analysis of change. Decade of behavior.* Washington, DC, US: American Psychological Association.

Collyer, C. E. (1986). Statistical techniques: Goodness-of-fit patterns in a computer cross-validation procedure comparing a linear and threshold model. *Behavior Research Methods, Instruments, & Computers, 18,* 618–622.

Cudeck, R., & Browne, M. W. (1983). Cross-validation of covariance structures. *Multivariate Behavioral Research, 18,* 147–157.

Diener, E., & Suh, E. M. (Eds.), (2000). *Culture and subjective well-being: Well being and quality of life.* Cambridge, MA: The MIT Press.

Embretson, S. E., & Reise, S. P. (2000). *Item response theory for psychologists.* Mahwah, NJ: Lawrence Erlbaum Associates.

Fisher, R. A. (1925). *Statistical methods for research workers.* Edinburgh: Oliver & Boyd.

Fisher, R. A. (1926). The arrangement of field experiments. *Journal of the ministry of agriculture of Great Britain, 33,* 505–513.

Fisher, R. A. (1935). *The design of experiments.* Edinburgh: Oliver & Boyd.

Gorsuch, R. L. (1983). *Factor Analysis* (second edition). Hillsdale, NJ: Lawrence Erlbaum Associates.

Grimm, L. G., & Yarnold, P. R. (1995). *Reading and understanding multivariate statistics.* Washington, DC: APA.

Grimm, L. G., & Yarnold, P. R. (2000). *Reading and understanding more multivariate statistics.* Washington, DC: APA.

Harlow, L. L., Mulaik, S. A., & Steiger, J. H. (1997). *What if there were no significance tests?* Mahwah, NJ: Lawrence Erlbaum Associates.

Hosmer, Jr., D. W., & Lemeshow, S. (2000). *Applied logistic regression.* New York, NY: John Wiley & Sons.

Jessor, R., & Jessor, S. L. (1973). A social psychology of marijuana use: Longitudinal studies of high school and college youth. *Journal of Personality and Social Psychology, 26,* 1–15.

Jöreskog, K. G. (1971). Simultaneous factor analysis in several populations. *Psychometrika, 57,* 409–426.

Kirk, R. E. (1996). Practical significance: A concept whose time has come. *Educational and Psychological Measurement, 56,* 746–759.

Kline, R. B. (2004). *Beyond significance testing: Reforming data analysis methods in behavioral research.* Washington, DC: American Psychological Association.

Lakoff, G., & Núñez, R. E. (2000). *Where mathematics comes from: How the embodied mind brings mathematics into being.* New York: Basic Books, A Member of the Perseus Books Groups.

Lord, F. M., & Novick, M. R. (1968). *Statistical theories of mental test scores.* Reading, MA: Addison-Wesley.

Marcoulides, G. A., & Hershberger, S. L. (1997). *Multivariate statistical methods: A first course.* Mahwah, NJ: Lawrence Erlbaum Associates.

Maxwell, S. E., & Delaney, H. D. (2004). *Designing experiments and analyzing data: A model comparison perspective.* Mahwah, NJ: Lawrence Erlbaum Associates.

McDonald, R. P. (1985). *Factor analysis and related methods.* Hillsdale, NJ: Lawrence Erlbaum Associates.

McDonald, R. P. (1997). Goodness of approximation in the linear model. In L. L. Harlow, S. A. Mulaik, & J. H. Steiger (Eds.), *What if there were no significance tests?* (pp. 199–219). Mahwah, NJ: Lawrence Erlbaum Associates.

McDonald, R. P. (1999). *Test theory: A unified treatment.* Mahwah, NJ: Lawrence Erlbaum Associates.

McDonald, R. P. (2000). A basis for multidimensional item response theory. *Applied Psychological Measurement, 24*, 99–114.

Meehl, P. E. (1997). The problem is epistemology, not statistics: Replace significance tests by confidence intervals and quantify accuracy of risky numerical predictions. In L. L. Harlow, S. A. Mulaik, & J. H. Steiger (Eds.), *What if there were no significance tests?* (pp. 393–425). Mahwah, NJ: Lawrence Erlbaum Associates.

Moskowitz, D. S., & Hershberger, S. L. (Eds.) (2002). *Modeling intraindividual variability with repeated measures data: Methods and applications.* Mahwah, NJ: Lawrence Erlbaum Associates.

Mulaik, S. A., Raju, N. S., & Harshman, R. A. (1997). A time and place for significance testing. In L. L. Harlow, S. A. Mulaik, & J. H. Steiger (Eds.), *What if there were no significance tests?* (pp. 65–115). Mahwah, NJ: Lawrence Erlbaum Associates.

Nash, J., with S. Nasar and H. W. Kuhn (Eds.) (2002). *The essential John Nash.* Princeton: Princeton University Press.

Pearl, J. (2000). *Causality: Models, reasoning and inference.* Cambridge, England: Cambridge University Press.

Pedhazur, E. J., & Schmelkin, L. P. (1991). *Measurement, design and analysis: An integrated approach.* Mahwah, NJ: Lawrence Erlbaum Associates.

Prochaska, J. O., & Velicer, W. F. (1997). The transtheoretical model of health behavior change. (Invited paper). *American Journal of Health Promotion, 12*, 38–48.

Rosenbaum, P. R. (2002). *Observational studies* (2nd ed.). New York: Springer Verlag.

Schmidt, F. L., & Hunter, J. E. (1997). Eight common but false objections to the discontinuation of significance testing in the analysis of research data. In L. L. Harlow, S. A. Mulaik, & J. H. Steiger (Eds.), *What if there were no significance tests* (pp. 37–64)? Mahwah, NJ: Lawrence Erlbaum Associates.

Shadish, W. R. (1995). The logic of generalization: Five principles common to experiments and ethnographies. *American Journal of Community Psychology, 23*, 419–428.

Shadish, W. R., Cook, T. D., & Campbell, D. T. (2002). *Experimental and quasi-experimental designs for generalized causal inference.* Boston: Houghton Mifflin Company.

Sörbom, D. (1974). A general method for studying difference in factor means and factor structures between groups. *British Journal of Mathematical and Statistical Psychology, 27*, 229–239.

Tabachnick, B. G., & Fidell, L. S. (2001). *Using multivariate statistics* (4th ed.). Boston: Allyn and Bacon.

Tatsuoka, M. M. (1970). *Discriminant analysis.* Champaign, IL: Institute for Personality and Ability Testing.

Tukey, J. W. (1953). *The problem of multiple comparisons.* Unpublished manuscript, Princeton University (mimeo).

Tukey, J. W. (1977). *Exploratory data analysis.* Reading, MA: Addison-Wesley.

Velicer, W. F., & Jackson, D. N. (1990). Component analysis versus common factor analysis: Some issues in selecting an appropriate procedure. *Multivariate Behavioral Research, 25*, 1–28.

Velicer, W. F., Prochaska, J. O., Fava, J. L., Rossi, J. S., Redding, C. A., Laforge, R. G., Robbins, M. L. (2000). Using the transtheoretical model for population-based approaches to health promotion and disease prevention. *Homeostasis in Health and Disease, 40*, 174–195.

Wheatley, M. J. (1994). *Leadership and the new science: Learning about organization from an orderly universe.* San Francisco, DA: Berrett-Koehler Publishers, Inc.

Wilkinson, L., & the APA Task Force on Statistical Inference (1999). Statistical methods in psychology journals: Guidelines and explanations. *American Psychologist, 54*, 594–604.

Wilks, S. S. (1932). Certain generalizations in the analysis of variance. *Biometrika, 24*, 471–494.

Wilson, E. O. (1998). *Consilience.* New York: Vintage Books, A division of Random House.

3

Background Themes

PRELIMINARY CONSIDERATIONS BEFORE MULTIVARIATE ANALYSES

Before addressing how the sets of themes relate specifically to a number of multivariate methods, it is helpful to notice several background themes that are essential to an understanding of quantitative methods, whether multivariate or univariate.

Devlin (1994) emphasizes that "abstract patterns are the very essence of thought, of communication, of computation, of society, and of life itself" (p. 7). The field of mathematics has long been concerned with noticing the fundamental patterns and connections in an area of study. In the more applied field of statistics, we can notice some basic themes that tend to permeate quantitative thinking. At least a preliminary understanding of them will help us later when delving into the complexities of specific multivariate methods.

Data

Data constitute the pieces of information (i.e., variables) on a phenomenon of interest. Data that can be assigned meaningful numerical values can be analyzed by a number of statistical methods. We usually assign a (numerical) score to each variable for each entity and store this in an "N by p" data matrix, where N stands for the number of participants or entities and p stands for the number of variables (predictors or outcomes). A data matrix is the starting point for statistical analysis. It is the large, numerical knowledge base from which we can combine, condense, and synthesize to derive meaningful and relevant statistical nuggets that capture the essence of the original information. Obviously, a data matrix will tend to have more columns (of variables) and most likely more rows (of participants) with multivariate research than with univariate methods. To the extent that the data are collected from a large and representative random sample, it can offer a strong foundation and workplace for subsequent analyses.

In later chapters, we examine a data matrix from 527 women at risk for HIV, examining a set of about 30 variables across three time points, measured 6 months apart. Thus, the full data set that is analyzed in this book is (N by p) $= 527$ by 90 and is a portion of a larger data collection that was funded by a grant from the National Institute of Mental Health (Harlow, Quina & Morokoff, 1991). At the end of each chapter that discusses a different multivariate method, we explore an example from this data set that addresses background themes and other considerations necessary when addressing a multivariate research question. The data, computer program setups, and analyses from these examples are presented in the accompanying CD.

Measurement Scales

Variables can be measured on a continuous or on a categorical scale. Variables measured on a continuous scale have numerical values that can be characterized by a smooth flow of arithmetically meaningful quantitative measurement, whereas categorical variables take on finite values that are discrete and more qualitatively meaningful. Age and height are examples of continuous variables that can take on many values that have quantitative meaning. In contrast, variables like gender and ethnicity have categorical distinctions that are not meaningfully aligned with any numerical values. It is also true that some variables can have measurement scales that have both numerical and categorical properties. Likert scale variables have several distinct categories that have at least ordinal, if not precisely quantitative, values. For example, variables that ask participants to rate a statement anywhere from "1 = strongly disagree" to "5 = strongly agree" are using an ordinal Likert scale of measurement.

Continuous variables can be used as either predictors or as outcomes (e.g., in multiple regression). Categorical variables are often used to separate people into groups for analysis with group-difference methods. For example, we may assign participants to a treatment or a control group with the categorical variable of treatment (with scores of 1 = 4 yes, or (0 = no). Because of the common use of Likert scales in social science research, the scale of such ordinal variables has been characterized as either categorical or quasi-continuous depending on whether the analysis calls for a grouping or a quantitative variable. As with any research decision, the conceptualization of a variable should be grounded in strong theoretical and empirical support.

As we will see later in this chapter, the choice of statistical analysis often depends, at least in part, on the measurement scales of the variables being studied. This is true for either multivariate or univariate methods. If variables are reliably and validly measured, whether categorical or continuous, then the results of analyses will be less biased and more trustworthy. We will also see that, before conducting multivariate methods, we often begin by analyzing frequencies on categorical data and examining descriptive statistics (e.g., means, standard deviations, skewness, and kurtosis) on continuous data. We will have a chance to do this in later chapters when providing the details from a fully worked-through example for each method.

Roles of Variables

Variables can be independent (i.e., perceived precipitating cause), dependent (i.e., perceived outcome), or mediating (i.e., forming a sequential link between independent and dependent variables). In research, it is useful to consider the role each variable plays in understanding phenomena. A variable that is considered a causal agent is sometimes labeled as independent or exogenous. It is not explained by a system of variables but is rather believed to have an effect on other variables. The affected variables are often referred to as dependent or endogenous, implying that they were directly impinged upon by other, more inceptive variables (e.g., Byrne, 2001).

Another kind of endogenous variable can be conceptualized as intermediate and thus intervenes between or changes the nature of the relationship between independent variables (IVs) and dependent variables (DVs). When a variable is conceived as a middle pathway between IVs and DVs it is often labeled as an intervening or mediating variable (e.g., Collins, Graham, & Flaherty, 1998; MacKinnon & Dwyer, 1993). For example, Schnoll, Harlow, Stolbach and Brandt (1998) found that the relationship between age, cancer stage, and psychological adjustment appeared to be mediated by coping style. In this model, age and cancer stage, the independent or exogenous variables, were not directly associated with psychological adjustment, the dependent or endogenous variable, after taking into account a cancer patient's coping style, the mediating (also endogenous) variable. Instead, cancer patients who were younger and had a less serious stage of cancer had more positive coping styles. Furthermore, those who coped more with a fighting spirit—rather than with hopelessness, fatalism, and anxious preoccupation—adjusted better. Thus, coping style served as a mediator between demographic/disease variables and psychological adjustment variables.

Variables are referred to as moderator variables when they change the nature of the relationship between the IVs and DVs variables (e.g., Baron & Kenny, 1986; Gogineni, Alsup, & Gillespie, 1995). For example, teaching style may be a predictor of an outcome, school performance. If another variable is identified, such as gender, that when multiplied by teaching style changes the nature of the predictive relationship, then gender is seen as a moderator variable. Thus, a moderator is an interaction formed between a hypothesized IV and another exogenous variable believed to have some effect on a DV when taken in conjunction with the first IV. In this example, we might find that teaching style is significantly related to school performance, whereas gender may not be related by itself. However, if an interaction is formed by multiplying the score for gender (e.g., 1 = male, 2 = female) by the teaching style score (e.g., 1 = lecture, 2 = interactive), we may find that this interaction is positively related to school performance. This would imply that individuals who are female and who are taught with an interactive teaching style are more apt to have higher school performance than other students. This finding suggests that gender moderated the relationship between teaching style and school performance (although we could just as easily state that teaching style moderated the relationship between gender and school performance, highlighting the importance of theory in hypothesis generation and interpretation of findings).

Moderating or mediating variables are also sometimes referred to as covariates. *Covariates* are variables that may correlate with a DV and are ideally *not* correlated with other IVs. Failing to consider covariates could hinder the interpretation of relationships between IVs and DVs, especially with nonrandom samples. Covariates help to statistically isolate an effect, especially when random assignment and/or manipulation are not accomplished. When several well-selected covariates (i.e., confounds, extraneous variables) are included in a study, and the relationship between the IVs and DVs still holds after controlling for the effects of one or more covariates, there is greater assurance that we have isolated the effect.

We should also realize that the designation of a variable as either independent, dependent, mediating, or moderating refers only to the role a variable plays within a specific research design. Using the variable psychological adjustment (Schnoll et al., 1998), we could assign it the role of IV (e.g., predictor of some outcome), mediator (e.g., intervening between some IV and a DV), moderator (e.g., part of an interaction between another variable, say gender, that is significantly related to a DV), or a DV (e.g., an outcome predicted by other IVs, mediators, and/or moderators). Ultimately, confirmation of a designated role is drawn from several sources of evidence (e.g., experimental design, longitudinal research, replication). Still, it is important to clearly articulate the intended role of variables in any design, hopefully with support and justification from previous theory and empirical research. Finally, we should realize that statistical methods can analyze multiple variables at a time, with multivariate methods allowing larger and more complex patterns of variables than other procedures.

Incomplete Information

Inherent in all statistical methods is the idea of analyzing incomplete information, where only a portion of knowledge is available. For example, we analyze a subset of the data by selecting a sample from the full population because this is all we have available to provide data. We examine only a subset of the potential causal agents or explaining variables, because it is nearly impossible to conceive of all possible predictors. We collect data from only a few measures for each variable of interest, because we do not want to burden our participants. We describe the main themes in the data (e.g., factors, dimensions) and try to infer past our original sample and measures to a larger population and set of constructs. In each case, there is a need to infer a generalizable outcome from a subset to a larger universe to explain how scores vary and covary. Ultimately, we would like to be able to demonstrate that associations among variables can be systematically explained with as little error as possible. For example, a researcher might find that alcohol use scores vary depending on the level of distress and the past history of alcohol abuse (Harlow, Mitchell, Fitts, & Saxon, 1999). It may be that the higher the level of distress and the greater the past history of substance abuse, the more likely someone is to engage in greater substance use. Strong designs and longitudinal data can help in drawing valid conclusions.

It is most likely true that other variables are important in explaining an outcome. Even when conducting a large, multivariate study, it is important to recognize that we cannot possibly examine the full set of information, largely because it is not usually known or accessible. Instead, we try to assess whether the pattern of variation and covariation in the data appears to demonstrate enough evidence for statistically significant relationships over and above what could be found from sheer random chance. Multivariate methods, much more so than univariable methods, offer more comprehensive procedures for analyzing real-world data that most likely have incomplete information.

Missing Data

Another background consideration is how to address missing data. Whether data are collected from an experiment or a survey, at least a portion of the participants invariably refrain from responding on some variables. If a sample is reasonably large (e.g., 200–400), the percent of missing data is small (e.g., 5% to 10%), and the pattern of missing data appears random, there are a number of options available. Although a thorough discussion of this topic is beyond the scope of this book, it is worth briefly describing several methods for approaching missing data.

Deleting data from all participants that have missing data is the most severe and probably one of the least preferable approaches to adopt. This method is called listwise deletion and can result in a substantially smaller data set, thus calling into question how representative the sample is of the larger population. I would not advise using this method unless there is a very large sample (e.g., 500 or more) and the percent of missing data is very small (i.e., <5%).

Pairwise deletion involves retaining most of the information from participants who have not provided complete data by dropping only the omitted data from a specific analysis. Thus, data from a participant we will call Jane may be missing for the variable self-esteem. We could still keep Jane's data on all other variables in an analysis and only drop her from calculations involving self-esteem. This approach results in having different sample sizes for different portions of an analysis, thereby providing questionable accuracy or stability.

Probably the most common method is to replace missing data with the mean from all of the complete data for a variable. Using the previous example, we could calculate the mean self-esteem score from all participants except Jane and then insert the mean for Jane's self-esteem score. This method yields an identical mean whether Jane's data is included or not. The standard deviation for mean-inserted data, however, is usually smaller and may not be an accurate indication of the variability in the population.

A wider range of missing data methods are currently discussed in the literature (Collins, Schafer, & Kam, 2001; Schafer, & Graham, 2002; Sijtsma, & van der Ark, 2003). One of these newer methods, multiple imputation, appears promising (Sinharay, Stern, & Russell, 2001) and has been successfully applied to multivariate methods, such as multiple regression (Enders, 2001). Multiple imputation involves inserting an estimate for the missing variable into several (e.g., 5 to 10) random subsets of the original data (Rubin, 2004). Analyses are then conducted on the multiple data sets and the results are averaged to provide more accurate parameter estimates. Calculating the standard deviation for the parameter estimate over the multiple datasets also provides a standard error that can be used to gauge the accuracy of the estimates. When the standard error is small, we have greater confidence in the accuracy of the parameter estimates.

Excellent discussions on missing data are available to interested readers (Allison, 2001; Cohen, Cohen, West, & Aiken, 2003; Little & Rubin, 2002; Rubin, 2004; Schafer & Schafer, 1997; Tabachnick & Fidell, 2001). We now turn to a brief discussion on descriptive statistics.

Descriptive Statistics

Descriptive statistics provide an ungirded view of data. This often involves summarizing the central nature of variables (e.g., average or mean score; midpoint or median score; and most frequently occurring or modal score), ideally from a representative sample. This also can comprise the spread or range of scores, as well as the average difference each score is from the mean (i.e., standard deviation). Descriptive statistics also can include measures of skewness, and kurtosis to indicate how asymmetric or lopsided, and how peaked or heavy-tailed, respectively, is a distribution of scores. Thus, descriptive statistics summarize basic characteristics of a distribution such as central tendency, variability, skewness, and kurtosis. Descriptive statistics can be calculated for large multivariate studies that investigate the relationships among a number of variables, hopefully based on a well-selected and large sample. With multivariate data, we organize the means from a set of variables in a column labeled a vector. We organize the variances and covariances among the variables into a variance-covariance matrix (see chapter 6).

Another form of descriptive statistics occurs when we synthesize information from multiple variables in a multivariate analysis using inferential statistics on a specific, nonrandom sample. For example, an instructor may want to describe the nature of class performance from a specific set of variables (e.g., quizzes, tests, projects, homework) and sample (e.g., one classroom). If she wanted to describe group differences between male and female students, she could conduct a multivariate analysis of variance with a categorical IV, gender, and the several continuous outcomes she measured from students' performance. Results would not necessarily be generalized beyond her immediate classroom, although they could provide a descriptive summary of the nature of performance between gender groups in her class of students.

Inferential Statistics

Inferential statistics allow us to generalize beyond our sample data to a larger population. With most statistical methods, inferences beyond one's specific data are more reliable when statistical assumptions are met.

Statistical assumptions for multivariate analyses include the use of representative samples, a normally or bell-shaped distribution of scores, linear relationships between the variables (i.e., variables that follow an additive pattern of the form: $Y = B_i X_i +$ error), and homoscedasticity (i.e., similar variance on one variable along all levels of another variable). We also would want to make sure that variables are not too highly overlapping or collinear. This would cause instability in statistical analyses so that it would be difficult to decide to which variable a weight should be attached. Generally, if variables are correlated greater than 0.90, collinearity is most likely present and decisions will have to be made as to whether to drop one of the variables or to combine them in a composite variable.

Examining skewness and kurtosis, bivariate plots of the variables, and correlations among the variables can check assumptions and collinearity. We also may want to consider whether any variables need to be transformed to meet assumptions. If any variables have skewness greater than an absolute value of about 1.0, or kurtosis greater than about 2.0, it may be helpful to consider taking a logarithmic transformation to reduce nonnormality. Although transformed scores are not in the original metric and interpretation may be difficult, many scores used in the social sciences have arbitrary scales. Thus, transformations, although somewhat controversial, still may be preferred to increase the power of analyses and decrease bias by meeting assumptions (Cohen, Cohen, West, & Aiken, 2003; Johnson & Wichern, 2002; Tabachnick & Fidell, 2001). Consider, making transformations especially when analyzing data concerned with extreme variables such as drug use and sexual risk. If the data can be transformed to meet assumptions, then inferences made on these data may be more accurate.

Inferential statistics allow estimates of population characteristics from samples representative of the population. Inferences are strengthened when potential extraneous variables are identified and taken into account. Likewise, if we can show that the data follow expected assumptions so that we can rule out random chance with our findings, then results are more conclusive. Multivariate research that shares these same features (i.e., representative samples, controlling for confounds, and normally distributed data) can provide a basis for inferences beyond the immediate sample to a large population of interest.

Roles of Variables and Choice of Methods

Although many statistical methods can be subsumed under a single, generalized linear model (McCullagh & Nelder, 1989), it is often useful to characterize different statistical methods by the roles played by the variables in an analysis.

Intermediate multivariate methods methods, such as multiple regression (MR) and analysis of covariance (ANCOVA) are more sophisticated than univariate methods (e.g., correlation, and analysis of variance: ANOVA). MR and ANCOVA are similar in that they both feature a single, continuous outcome variable and two or more IVs, at least one of which is continuous. They differ in that variables for MR (i.e., the multiple IVs and single outcome) are often all continuous. In contrast, ANCOVA always has at least one categorical IV, much like ANOVA. ANCOVA differs from ANOVA in that ANCOVA has both continuous and categorical IVs, allowing the use of continuous covariates as well as grouping IV(s) to help explain the single outcome variable.

Categorical or grouping multivariate methods such as multivariate analysis of variance (MANOVA), discriminant function analysis (DFA), and logistic regression (LR) allow an examination of the links between a set of variables and a set of categories or groups. MANOVA is an extension of ANOVA, allowing multiple, continuous DVs and one or more categorical IVs that each have two or more groups. Variables used in DFA have the same characteristics as those with MANOVA except that the roles are reversed. In DFA, the set of continuous variables is viewed as predictor variables and the set of groups is seen as aspects of a categorical outcome variable. When there is a mixture of both categorical and continuous predictors and a categorical outcome, LR is often used. DFA and LR are very similar in the nature and roles for the variables, with some differences. DFA requires multivariate assumptions (e.g., normality, linearity, and homoscedasticity), whereas LR does not. Further, DFA focuses on standardized or structure weights that can be interpreted much like correlation coefficients between a continuous predictor and the categorical outcome. In LR, weights are interpreted as the odds that an individual with the IV characteristic will end up in a specific outcome group (Hosmer & Lemeshow, 2000). If there is a 50/50 chance of ending up in a specific group, the odds will be equal to 1.0. If there is less chance, then the odds will be less than 1.0; conversely, if there is greater than a 50/50 chance of being in a specific group based on the IV characteristic, the odds will be greater than 1.0. Predictor variables that are meaningful in an analysis generally have an odds value different from 1.0 associated with them.

Multivariate correlational methods, such as canonical correlation (CC), principal components analysis (PCA), and factor analysis (FA) incorporate a large set of continuous variables. In CC, there are two sets of variables, where the goal is to explore the patterns of relationships between the two sets (see Chapter 10). In PCA or FA, there is one set of continuous variables with the goal of trying to identify a smaller set of latent dimensions that underlie the variables (see Chapter 11).

Summary of Background Themes

Multivariate statistical methods build on these background themes allowing more realistic designs among multiple variables than methods that just analyze one (i.e., univariate) or two (i.e., bivariate) key variables. Multivariate methods can help us see relationships that might only occur in combination with a set of well-selected variables.

Background themes involve consideration of the data used to test the hypotheses, the scale of measurement and the nature of the variables, both descriptive and inferential statistics, and how the scale of the variables often affects the choice of method (e.g., intermediate, categorical or grouping multivariate, or correlational multivariate) for a particular study. A summary of background themes to consider for multivariate methods is presented in Table 3.1.

TABLE 3.1
Summary of Background Themes to Consider for Multivariate Methods

a. Data matrix (N rows of participants and p columns of variables)
b. Measurement scales (categorical or continuous)
c. Types of variables (independent, dependent, mediating, or moderating)
d. Incomplete information (analyze only a subset)
e. Descriptive statistics (central tendency, variability, skewness, and kurtosis)
f. Inferential statistics (requiring assumptions to generalize beyond the sample)
g. Types of variables and choice of methods (intermediate methods with one continuous DV; multivariate group difference methods; and multivariate correlational methods)

QUESTIONS TO HELP APPLY THEMES TO MULTIVARIATE METHODS

Having considered a number of themes that enhance multivariate thinking, it is instructive to briefly outline how these themes apply to several multivariate methods. To do this in the upcoming chapters, it is helpful to reflect on a set of questions to ask. These questions can help us focus on how the major themes apply to various statistical procedures. My hope is that, by working through a set of relevant questions on several multivariate statistics, it will be much easier to extend this thinking to other methods not discussed in this volume.

Thus, the main focus of this book is not to present complete details on every multivariate method. Rather, I present a set of themes and questions to help enlarge our thinking to recognize the common facets of many statistical methods. In keeping with Devlin's (1994) claim that "most mathematicians now agree [that] mathematics is the science of patterns" (p. 3), I argue that multivariate statistics embody a set of prevalent ideas or propositions. To the extent that these elemental ideas are apparent, it is much easier to engage in multivariate thinking.

The first question to ask is, What is this method and how is it similar to and different from other methods? For each method, a brief description of the main features is presented. I then point to other methods that are similar to, and different from, the particular method being discussed, thereby inviting an initial understanding of the connections among methods.

A second question I ask is, When is this method used and what research questions can it address? In this section I present a few common uses of the specific multivariate method, often providing brief examples. Information presented in this section can help when trying to decide which method to use for a particular research hypothesis.

The third question asks, What are the main multiplicity themes for this method? Because the notion of multiplicity tends to pervade all multivariate methods, this section can start to sound repetitive when working through the various procedures presented in this volume. Nonetheless, this reiteration helps deepen and widen understanding of the scope and capabilities of multivariate methods. Readers can refer back to Chapter 2 to refresh themselves with each of the multiplicity themes, when needed.

A fourth question is, What are the main background themes applied to this method? I work through much of the discussion in this Chapter for each method, explicating several considerations that are important to attend to before conducting the main multivariate analyses.

The fifth question asked is, What is the statistical model that is tested with this method? The topic of models can appear obscure and abstract. It is helpful to think of a model as a concise representation of a large system or phenomenon (Britt, 1997). Thus, a model is just an abbreviated description. To the extent that a model is quantified, it becomes more capable of being examined and tested in a rigorous, scientific arena. I like to think of a progression of models from a verbal or conceptual description, to symbolic and pictorial representation (as in a flow chart or path diagram), to one or more mathematical equations. Many statistical methods can be accommodated under what is known as the generalized linear model (McCullagh, & Nelder, 1989), showing how a variable is an additive linear combination of other constants or variables. For example, in basic mathematics, a straight line is modeled as $Y = A + BX$, where Y is an outcome variable, A is a (constant) point at which a line intersects with the Y axis, B is the (constant) slope of a line (i.e., rise over run), and X is a predictor or independent variable. This simple linear formulation emerges in each of the multivariate models presented in this volume.

A sixth question asks, How do central themes of variance, covariance, and linear combinations apply? These central themes, discussed in Chapter 2, get at the heart of statistics. We are reminded that much of science seeks to explain and predict how variables vary and covary, recognizing that large sets of variables may have to be summarized in linear combinations.

The seventh question is, What are the main themes needed to interpret results at a macro-level? To aid with interpretation, it is useful to examine results at a global, overriding level, often with a test of significance and a measure of the magnitude of an effect. For each multivariate method presented here, a macro-level approach is described and then applied with real-world data.

Similarly, question eight asks, What are the main themes needed to interpret results at a micro-level? This section suggests how to understand the specific aspects of a multivariate analysis, often focusing on some description of means or correlational weights.

A ninth question is, What are some other considerations or next steps after applying this method? Here, we examine ways to follow up a multivariate analysis, recognizing that any single finding is just one portion of the larger body of knowledge in a field of study.

Question 10 asks, What is an example of applying this method to a research question? For each multivariate method presented in this volume, we work through an example using a consistent data set (included on the accompanying CD).

Table 3.2 presents a summary of the 10 questions.

Finally, each chapter that presents a multivariate method ends with a summary chart that outlines how the major themes apply. For example, most methods benefit from considering multiplicity themes of multiple theories, hypotheses, empirical studies, controls, time points, samples, and measures. Similarly, most methods gain from careful attention to background themes concerning data, measurement, assumptions, and inferences. Likewise, most methods focus to some degree on the central themes of variance, covariance, and ratios of (co-)variances.

Questions to ask when addressing interpretation themes are provided for each of the methods. Responses to each question provide an integrated presentation

TABLE 3.2
Questions to Ask for Each Multivariate Method

1. What is this method and how is it similar to and different from other methods?
2. When is this method used and what research questions can it address?
3. What are the main multiplicity themes for this method?
4. What are the main background themes applied to this method?
5. What is the statistical model that is tested with this method?
6. How do central themes of variance, covariance, and linear combinations apply?
7. What are the main themes needed to interpret results at a macro-level?
8. What are the main themes needed to interpret results at a micro-level?
9. What are some other considerations or next steps after applying this method?
10. What is an example of applying this method to a research question?

of common and unique aspects for a number of multivariate methods, hopefully helping to demystify these procedures and encourage their wider application.

REFERENCES

Allison, P. D. (2001). *Missing data (Quantitative Applications in the Social Sciences)*. Newbury Park, CA: Sage.

Baron, R. M., & Kenny, D. A. (1986). The moderator-mediator variable distinction in social psychological research: Conceptual, strategic, and statistical considerations. *Journal of Personality and Social Psychology, 51,* 1173–1182.

Britt, D. W. (1997). *A conceptual introduction to modeling: Qualitative and quantitative perspectives.* Mahwah, NJ: Lawrence Erlbaum Associates.

Byrne, B. M. (2001). *Structural Equation Modeling with AMOS: Basic Concepts, Applications, and Programming.* Mahwah, NJ: Lawrence Erlbaum Associates.

Cohen, J., Cohen, P., West, S. G., & Aiken, L. S. (2003). *Applied multiple regression/correlation analysis for behavioral sciences* (3rd ed.). Mahwah, NJ: Lawrence Erlbaum Associates.

Collins, L. M., Graham, J. W., & Flaherty, B. P. (1998). An alternative framework for defining mediation. *Multivariate Behavioral Research, 33,* 295–312.

Collins, L. M., Schafer, J. L., Kam, C. M. (2001). A comparison of inclusive and restrictive strategies in modern missing data procedures. *Psychological Methods, 6*(4), 330–351.

Devlin, K. (1994). *Mathematics: The science of patterns. The search for order in life, mind, and the universe.* New York: Scientific American Library.

Enders, C. K. (2001). The performance of the full information maximum likelihood estimator in multiple regression models with missing data. *Educational & Psychological Measurement, 61,* 713–740.

Gogineni, A., Alsup, R., & Gillespie, D. F. (1995). Mediation and moderation in social work research. *Social Work Research, 19,* 57–63.

Harlow, L. L., Mitchell, K. J., Fitts. S. N., & Saxon, S. E. (1999). Psycho-existential distress and problem behaviors: Gender, subsample and longitudinal tests. *Journal of Applied Biobehavioral Reasearch, 4,* 111–138.

Harlow, L. L., Quina, K., & Morokoff, P. (1991). *Predicting heterosexual HIV-risk in women.* NIMH Grant MH47233 (awarded $500,000).

Hosmer, D. W., & Lemeshow, S. (2000). *Applied logistic regression* (2nd ed.). New York: Wiley.

Johnson, R. A., & Wichern, D. W. (2002). *Applied multivariate statistical analysis* (2nd ed.). Englewood Cliffs, NJ: Prentice-Hall, Inc.

Little, R. J. A., & Rubin, D. B. (2002). *Statistical analysis with missing data* (2nd ed.). New York: Wiley.

MacKinnon, D. P., & Dwyer, J. H. (1993). Estimating mediated effects in prevention studies. *Evaluation Review, 17*(2), 144–158.

McCullagh, P., & Nelder, J. A. (1989). *Generalized linear models* (2nd ed.). London: Chapman & Hall.

Rubin, D. B. (2004). *Multiple imputation for nonresponse in surveys.* New York: Wiley.

Schafer, J. L., & Schafer, J. (1997). *Analysis of incomplete multivariate data.* London: Chapman & Hall/CRC.

Schnoll, R. A., Harlow, L. L., Stolbach, L. L., & Brandt, U. (1998). A structural model of the relationships among disease, age, coping, and psychological adjustment in women with breast cancer. *Psycho-Oncology, 7*, 69–77.

Sijtsma, K., & van der Ark, L. A. (2003). Investigation and treatment of missing item scores in test and questionnaire data. *Multivariate Behavioral Research, 38*, 505–528.

Sinharay, S., Stern, H. S., & Russell, D. (2001). The use of multiple imputation for the analysis of missing data. *Psychological Methods, 6*, 317–329.

Tabachnick, B. G., & Fidell, L. S. (2001). *Using multivariable statistics* (4th ed.). Boston: Allyn and Bacon.

II

Intermediate Multivariate Methods With 1 Continuous Outcome

4

Multiple Regression

Themes Applied to Multiple Regression (MR)

Having considered a number of themes that run through multivariate methods, it is instructive to view how these themes apply to MR. To do this, the set of 10 questions presented in the previous chapter are outlined with discussion on how to respond to them if considering the use of MR in a research study. MR can be considered an intermediate method that highlights some of the complexities of correlational methods that allow for more than one independent variable (IV). MR also serves as a foundation to develop and comprehend other more extensive methods.

WHAT IS MR AND HOW IS IT SIMILAR TO AND DIFFERENT FROM OTHER METHODS?

MR is a prediction statistic that allows us to have two or more IVs and one dependent variable (DV) or criterion. Typically, the variables are all continuous, although MR can handle other kinds of variables. If our main research question involves predicting a single outcome from a set of relevant predictors or IVs, then MR would be a useful method to consider. MR can be classified as an intermediate method, somewhere between the bivariate methods of correlation and linear regression and multivariate methods such as canonical correlation (see Chapter 10). It differs from correlation and linear regression in that MR has more than one IV. It differs from canonical correlation in that MR is limited to just a single outcome or DV. MR differs from other predictive methods of discriminant function analysis (DFA) and logistic regression (LR) because both DFA and LR are used with a categorical outcome. We will discuss more about DFA and LR methods in Chapters 8 and 9, respectively.

For those who are interested in a very thorough and readable presentation of MR, consider the acclaimed volume *Applied Multiple Regression/Correlation Analysis for the Behavioral Sciences* (3rd ed.), by Cohen, Cohen, West and Aiken (2003).

WHEN IS MR USED AND WHAT RESEARCH QUESTIONS CAN IT ADDRESS?

Although there are several kinds of regression procedures (e.g., logit, nonlinear, polynomial, and set), discussion here is limited to three common approaches to MR; each used in different circumstances:

a. **Standard MR**. This approach loads all predictors in one step. It is useful when predicting or explaining a single phenomenon with a set of predictors (e.g., predict amount of condom use with a set of attitudinal, interpersonal and behavioral variables). Figure 4.1 depicts this example with three predictors.

b. **Hierarchical MR**. This form, also called sequential MR, allows researchers to theoretically order variables in specific steps. It allows assessment of whether a set of variables substantially adds to prediction, over and above one or more other variables already in the analysis (e.g., assess whether attitudinal variables increase prediction, over and above behavioral predictors of condom use).

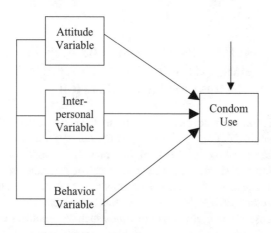

FIG. 4.1. Depiction of standard MR with three predictors, where the lines connecting the three IVs depict correlations among predictors and the arrow headed toward the outcome variable represents prediction error.

c. **Stepwise MR**. This kind, sometimes called statistical MR, has the computer select variables for entry. Selection is based on the IV that has the strongest partial correlation with the DV, after controlling for the effect of variables already in the equation. This form capitalizes on chance variation in the data much more than standard or hierarchical MR, and for this reason it is not often recommended (Cohen, Cohen, West, & Aiken, 2003). Still, it may be useful when it is important to identify the most salient predictors of an outcome, particularly in a new field that does not allow much theory to guide the researcher. For example, a researcher could assess which are the most important predictors (i.e., behavioral, attitudinal, or environmental) of an outcome variable designating a new form of disease. Because of the atheoretical nature of stepwise MR, a large sample size and replication should be used.

WHAT ARE THE MAIN MULTIPLICITY THEMES FOR MR?

As with most multivariate methods, the theme of multiplicity is pervasive in the effective use of MR. Before conducting a MR analysis, a thoughtful review of the literature and thinking in an area of study should reveal one or more pertinent theories. Theory would help in directing all aspects of an analysis, beginning with research hypotheses that would most likely involve statements about prediction, to the choice of multiple, continuous IVs and a single, continuous DV, to a consideration of previous empirical research. We also would want to consider collecting data from multiple, representative samples to replicate and generalize findings past the initial group of participants. Finally, we also may want to look into the use of multiple time points and multiple controls, especially if we wanted to build causal evidence about the direction and magnitude of causation. Multiple time points could be incorporated by using variables collected at the first time point, $t1$, as predictors, and a single outcome variable collected at $t2$. We include multiple controls by having several well-selected confounding or covariate variables that may be related to the DV, although they are not the central focus. If the main variable(s) showed significant correlation with the outcome, over and above correlation among the confounding variables and the outcome, there would be some evidence for isolating the relationship between the IV(s) and DV.

WHAT ARE THE MAIN BACKGROUND THEMES APPLIED TO MR?

Background themes can be applied to MR to help us begin to understand how to use this popular method. A large ($N \times p$) data set would be needed, allowing for multiple IVs and a single DV. With six or more predictors, sample size should be at least 100 (Green, 1991), and much more (e.g., 200–400+) when assumptions are violated or when capitalizing on chance variation (e.g., with stepwise MR). We also should compute descriptive statistics (e.g., means, standard deviations) and test assumptions (i.e., examine bivariate scatter plots for pairs of variables, and skewness and kurtosis for all variables).

If data do not appear to conform to assumptions (e.g., normality, linearity), consider making transformations on pertinent variables. For example, a variable such as substance abuse could be highly lopsided to the left (i.e., positively skewed). This would indicate that most individuals reported low or no substance abuse, whereas a few individuals reported moderate to high substance use. This pattern of responses would be depicted by a peak at the low end of the score range with a tail trailing off to the right or high end of the range of scores. In this case, it would be helpful to consider transforming the scores to readjust the variable into one that more closely followed assumptions (e.g., normality). Several transformations could be considered (e.g., logarithm or square root) to assess which is best for evening out the distribution of a variable such as substance abuse. Several excellent discussions of transformations are offered elsewhere (Cohen, Cohen, West & Aiken, 2003; Tabachnick & Fidell, 2001).

Correlations among the variables and reliability coefficients also should be calculated at this point. Because MR assumes that predictors are perfectly reliable, regression coefficients are biased with unreliable variables. To the extent that data were randomly selected and relevant, the data met assumptions, and predictors are reasonably reliable (e.g., reliability coefficients ≥ 0.70), we could infer past the initial sample to a larger population with some degree of confidence. Correlations also should be scanned to ensure that variables are not overly correlated (i.e., multicollinear) with other variables. Correlations of 0.90 or higher indicate clear multicollinearity, although correlations as high as 0.70 may be suggestive of a potential problem (Tabachnick & Fidell, 2001).

WHAT IS THE STATISTICAL MODEL THAT IS TESTED WITH MR?

In MR, we begin by summarizing a set of independent (X) variables with a linear combination, which can be labeled, X' so that:

$$X' = A + B1(X1) + B2(X2) + B3(X3) + \cdots + Bp(Xp) \qquad (4.1)$$

where A = a constant or Y-intercept, Bi = an unstandardized regression weight or constant that indicates how much an outcome (Y) variable would change if the X variable were changed by one unit, and p = the number of predictors. The linear combination of X scores, X', is selected so that it has the least squared distance from the outcome Y scores. We can then depict a model in which the outcome variable, Y, is seen as a function of this linear combination of the X variables, X', plus some prediction error, E, that represents variance that is not related to any of the X variables. Thus, the model for MR could be written as:

$$Y = X' + E \qquad (4.2)$$

The goal is to find the multiple correlation, R, between X' and Y and show that it is significantly different from zero. Significance tests for individual regression weights, B, are then conducted to determine which of the independent (X) variables significantly predict the outcome variable, Y. Seen in this way, a MR model is very similar to a model between just a single X and a single Y variable. The main difference is that with MR, the single predictor, X', is actually a linear combination of multiple X variables.

HOW DO CENTRAL THEMES OF VARIANCE, COVARIANCE, AND LINEAR COMBINATIONS APPLY TO MR?

In MR, variance can refer to the amount of shared variance (i.e., R^2) between the best linear combination of the X variables (X') and Y. Variance also can refer to the amount of nonoverlapping or prediction error variance (i.e., $1 - R^2$) between X' and Y. For both of these, we are actually looking at how much X' covaries with Y, relative to how much variance there is in X' and Y, separately. We also look at the ratio of explained variance over unexplained variance for the F-test:

$$F = (R^2/\text{p})/[(1 - R^2)/(N - \text{p} - 1)] \qquad (4.3)$$

that is tested on p and $N - \text{p} - 1$ degrees of freedom. In MR (Cohen, Cohen, West, & Aiken, 2003), we can use R^2 to examine how much variance is shared between the linear combination of predictors and the single outcome variable. As we see in the next section, we can also use R^2 as an indication of the magnitude of the effect in MR.

WHAT ARE THE MAIN THEMES NEEDED TO INTERPRET RESULTS AT A MACRO-LEVEL?

Whenever interpreting a MR analysis, the first step would be to assess whether there was statistical significance at the omnibus or macro level. This is not too much different from examining an omnibus F-test in analysis of variance (ANOVA) before looking for more specific information in planned comparisons.

Correlational methods such as MR make use of an F-test to assess whether the covariance among variables is significantly larger than chance relative to the variance within variables (see Chapter 1 for more discussion of this). When the value of an F-test is significantly large (as deemed by appropriate statistical tables[1]), we can conclude that there is sufficient evidence of relationships occurring at the macro-level. The F-test examines whether the degree of association, as indicated by R (i.e., multiple R) is significantly greater than zero. Multiple R provides a measure of overall association between the best linear combination of the IV predictors, X', and the single DV, Y. In MR, the method of forming the linear combination, which is called least squares, maximizes the value for multiple R, the correlation between X' and Y. Because a whole set of variables are combined, some of which may relate negatively and others relate positively with the outcome, multiple R can take on values only from 0 to 1.0 and cannot have negative values. It is interpreted as in bivariate correlation, r, with values closer to 1.0 indicating stronger association. An indication of the direction of prediction is gleaned from the sign associated with the individual regression weights.

Effect sizes provide an indication of the magnitude of our findings. They are a useful supplement to a significance test (Cohen, 1992). Effect size (ES) calculations for MR are often proportions of shared variance (Cohen, 1988, 1992; Kirk, 1996). Similar to r^2 in bivariate regression, Multiple R^2 gives the proportion of variance in the DV that can be explained by the (linear combination of) IVs. It is useful by providing a single number that conveys how much the scores from a set of variables (co-)vary in the same way (i.e., rise and fall together), relative to how much the scores within each variable differ among themselves. R^2 is also a measure of multivariate or macro-level effect size. As suggested by Cohen (1992), a R^2 of 0.02 represents a small multivariate ES; 0.13 is a medium ES, and 0.26 is a large ES. An adjusted R^2 is sometimes calculated to adjust for sample size and the number of predictors, providing a more accurate estimate of the population R^2 value:

$$\text{Adjusted } R^2 = 1 - (1 - R^2)(N - 1)/(N - p - 1) \qquad (4.4)$$

There is less adjustment with a large sample size, N, and a small number of predictors, p. The adjusted R^2 value could be substantially smaller than the original R^2 with a small sample size and a large number of predictors. The example provided at the end of the chapter provides a calculation for an adjusted R^2 value with a sample size of 527 and four predictors. As can be expected, there is very little adjustment with such a large sample size and only a few predictors.

---

[1] Also see the webpage: http://members.aol.com/johnp71/pdfs.html to calculate F, t, z, and X^2 values or corresponding p values.

WHAT ARE THE MAIN THEMES
NEEDED TO INTERPRET RESULTS
AT A MICRO-LEVEL?

After determining that the least squares linear combination of X variables, X', is significantly related to the outcome variable, Y, we can then investigate which variables are contributing to the overall relationship. As with macro-level assessment, we first examine statistical tests and then proceed to evaluate the magnitude of the effects.

Significance t-Tests for Variables

In MR, we can examine the significance of each independent variable by t-tests. We may want to set a conservative level of alpha (e.g., $p < 0.01$) for t-tests or even consider using a Bonferroni approach. The latter approach establishes a set alpha level (e.g., $p = 0.05$) and then distributes the available alpha level over the number of t-tests conducted (i.e., p or the number of predictors). Thus, if there were four predictors and a desired alpha level of 0.05, each predictor could be evaluated with a p value of 0.0125 or some unequal portion of p across t-tests.

Weights

After determining that a variable is a significant predictor of Y, we usually want to examine the standardized weights that indicate how much a specific variable is contributing to an analysis. In MR, we examine least squares regression weights that tell us how much a predictor variable covaries with an outcome variable after taking into account the relationships with other predictor variables. Thus, a standardized regression coefficient is a partial correlation between a specific predictor, Xi, and the Y, that does not include the correlation between Xi and the other X variables. The standardized regression weight, or beta weight, β, indicates the relationship between a predictor and the outcome, after recognizing the correlations among the other predictor variables in the equation. High absolute values ($\geq |0.30|$) indicate better predictive value for standardized regression coefficients.

In an unstandardized metric (i.e., B), the weight represents the change in an outcome variable that can be expected when a predictor variable is changed by one unit. We could focus on the unstandardized regression weights for at least two reasons. The first is when we want to assess the significance of a predictor variable. To do this, we examine the ratio of the unstandardized regression weight over the standard error associated with a specific variable, forming a critical ratio that is interpreted as a t-test. If the p-value associated with the t-test is greater than a designated level (e.g., 0.05 or 0.01), then the variable is said to be a significant predictor of the outcome variable. The second reason to focus on unstandardized regression coefficients is if we want to compare regression weights with those from another sample or form a prediction equation for possible use in another sample. The unstandardized regression weights retain the original metric and provide a better basis for comparing across different samples that may have different standardized weights even when unstandardized weights are similar (Pedhazur, 1997).

Regression weights can also provide a measure of ES. To keep the micro-level ES in the same metric as the macro-level R^2, we could square the standardized β coefficients. Much like values for bivariate r^2, values of β^2 could be interpreted as small, medium, and large micro-level ESs when equal to 0.01, 0.06, and 0.13, respectively.

Squared Semipartial Correlations

These represent the change in R^2 at a particular step in the equation. A squared semipartial correlation can be viewed as a unique effect size for a specific variable, after taking into account other variables that are already predicting Y. We calculate this value by subtracting the value of R^2 obtained from a smaller set of predictors, from the R^2 obtained from a larger set of predictors. Thus, if R^2 is 0.25 with three predictors and increases to 0.32 when adding a fourth predictor, the squared semipartial correlation for $X4$ would be $(0.32 - 0.25 = 0.07)$, which would indicate a small to medium unique effect size.

WHAT ARE SOME OTHER CONSIDERATIONS OR NEXT STEPS AFTER APPLYING MR?

After conducting a MR and finding a significant macro effect (i.e., the F-test reveals that R^2 is significantly different from zero), and several significant predictors (i.e., t-tests are significant for the regression coefficients), we may want to consider whether we can generalize past the initial sample. If possible, it is helpful to replicate and cross-validate findings, possibly with a different method such as an experimental design, or a longitudinal study design to verify temporal ordering. Reliability of variables should be reconsidered and variables should be improved, when possible. Finally, it is important to consider whether sufficient confounds were included so that the main variables were isolated in the MR. That is, were other variables included in the MR analysis to assess whether the hypothesized relationships between the main IVs and the DV still held when taking possible extraneous variables into account? For example, if predicting condom use from attitudinal, interpersonal, and behavioral variables (see example in Figure 4.1), would adding frequency of sex as a potential confound lessen the degree of relationship between the original three predictors and the outcome? If not, then we can rule out frequency of sex as a confound, thereby strengthening the validity of the relationships found.

WHAT IS AN EXAMPLE OF APPLYING MR TO A RESEARCH QUESTION?

An example provides a clearer view of how to apply MR to real-word data. Analyses draw on theories of the transtheoretical model (Prochaska & Velicer, 1997) and the multifaceted model of HIV risk (Harlow, Quina, Morokoff, Rose, & Grimley, 1993). The hypothesized outcome is stage of condom use (STAGE), with higher values indicating greater frequency and a longer time period of (readiness for) using condoms. Thus, values were assigned so that, $1 =$ precontemplation (i.e., not thinking about condom use), $2 =$ contemplation (i.e., considering condom use), $3 =$ preparation (i.e., taking initial steps such as buying condoms to use), $4 =$ action (i.e., using condoms for up to 6 months), and $5 =$ maintenance (i.e., consistently using condoms for more than 6 months). A set of four predictors was selected: pros of condom use (PROS), cons of condom use (CONS), self-efficacy for condom use (CONSEFF), and psychosexual functioning (PSYSX). Data were collected at three time points, 6 months apart. In the descriptions below, the designation of a specific time point is made by adding "A" at the end of variable collected at an initial time point, "B" for variables collected 6 months later, and "C" to indicate variables collected 1 year after baseline. MR analyses use data collected at the "B" time point.

Based on previous empirical literature (Goldman & Harlow, 1993; Harlow, Rose, Morokoff, Quina, Mayer, Mitchell, & Schnoll, 1998; Marcus, Eaton, Rossi, & Harlow, 1994; Prochaska et al., 1994a, b), I conducted several analyses on data from 527 women at risk for HIV (see Harlow et al., 1998). Below is SAS (1999) computer output in Tables 4.1 to 4.19 with brief comments for this example, regarding the following: descriptive statistics, reliability and correlations, standard MR, hierarchical MR, and stepwise MR.

Descriptive Statistics

Notice from the descriptive statistics of Table 4.1 that all the variables are relatively normally distributed. Skewness values are within an acceptable range of -1.0 to $+1.0$, except for PROSB, which shows slight skewness. Kurtosis values are all reasonable (i.e., below 2.0), indicating that the data are not all piled up at specific values.

TABLE 4.1
Descriptive Statistics for 4 IVs and the DV, Stage of Condom Use

Variable	Mean	SD	Min	Max	Skewness	Kurtosis
PROSB	4.07	0.81	1.00	5.00	-1.05	0.93
CONSB	2.05	0.84	1.00	5.00	0.89	0.49
CONSEFFB	3.51	1.15	1.00	5.00	-0.45	-0.82
PSYSXB	4.01	0.75	1.67	5.00	-0.66	-0.13
STAGEB	2.44	1.38	1.00	5.00	0.79	-0.61

TABLE 4.2
Coefficient Alpha and Test-Retest Reliability Coefficients

		Time Points		
Variable	*Coefficient Alpha*	*A and B*	*B and C*	*A and C*
PROS	0.81	0.60	0.65	0.55
CONS	0.83	0.61	0.63	0.58
CONSEFF	0.89	0.62	0.63	0.55
PSYSX	0.85	0.66	0.68	0.60
STAGE	—	0.67	0.69	0.63

Reliability Coefficients and Correlations

Six-month test–retest reliabilities, shown in Table 4.2, are at least 0.60, indicating relative stability across an extended time. Coefficient alpha values are greater than 0.80 for the four multi-item variables, indicating high internal consistency.

Correlations among the four predictors (PROSB, CONSB, CONSEFFB, and PSYSXB) and the outcome variable (STAGEB) show low to moderate relationships (see Table 4.3). There is no concern with collinearity, because no correlation, particularly among IVs, approaches problem levels of 0.70 to 0.90.

Standard Multiple Regression
(DV: STAGEB)

The F-test (see calculations, below, and Table 4.4) indicate that Y and the best least-squares combination of the predictor variables, X', are correlated significantly

TABLE 4.3
Correlation Coefficients Within Time B, $N = 527$

		Probabilities $> |r|$ *with* H0$:\rho = 0$			
	PROSB	*CONSB*	*CONSEFFB*	*PSYSXB*	*STAGEB*
PROSB	1.000	−0.169	0.361	0.058	0.263
		<0.0001	<0.0001	0.1806	<0.0001
CONSB	−0.169	1.000	−0.489	−0.320	−0.315
	<0.0001		<0.0001	<0.0001	<0.0001
CONSEFFB	0.361	−0.489	1.000	0.239	0.447
	<0.0001	<0.0001		<0.0001	<0.0001
PSYXB	0.058	−0.320	0.239	1.000	−0.103
	0.1806	<0.0001	<0.0001		0.0177
STAGEB	0.263	−0.315	0.447	−0.103	1.000
	<0.0001	<0.0001	<0.0001	0.0177	

TABLE 4.4
Summary of Macro-Level Standard MR Output

| | | Analysis of Variance | | | |
Source	df	Sum of Squares	Mean Square	F-Value	Prob. > F
Model	4	287.068	71.76703	52.28	<0.0001
Error	522	716.552	1.37271		
Corrected total	526	1003.620			
Root MSE		1.17163	R-Square		0.2860
Dependent Mean		2.43643	Adjusted R^2		0.2806
Coeff Var		48.08773			

different from zero. The multivariate effect size, R^2, is large (i.e., >0.26), as is the adjusted R^2 (see below) that corrects for sample size and the number of predictors.

Using equation 4.3, presented earlier, we could verify the value for the F-test by showing that $F(4,522) = (R^2/p)/(1 - R^2)/(N - p - 1) = (0.286/4)/(0.714)/(527 - 4 - 1) = 0.0715/0.001368 = 52.27$.

Note that Table 4.4 also presents a value for adjusted R^2 that provides an indication of the true value of R^2 in the population. The value for adjusted R^2 is very close to the unadjusted value because of the large sample size and the relatively small number of predictors. The adjusted R^2 value would be markedly less than the unadjusted value with small sample sizes and a large number of predictors. For our example, the value for adjusted R^2 could be verified by solving for Equation 4.4:

$$\text{Adjusted } R^2 = 1 - (1 - R^2)(N - 1)/(N - p - 1)$$
$$= 1 - 0.714(526/522) = 1 - 0.714(1.00766) = 0.2805$$

Table 4.5 presents a micro-level summary of the regression coefficients for the standard MR. Examining the unstandardized weights (i.e., parameter estimates) and their associated t-values, we see that all the predictors are significantly related to stage of readiness to use condoms (i.e., STAGEB). Combining Equations 4.1

TABLE 4.5
Summary of Micro-Level Standard MR Output

| | | Parameter Estimates | | | | |
Variable	df	Parameter Estimate	Standard Error	t-value	Prob. > |t|	Standardized Estimate
Intercept	1	2.705	0.473	5.72	<0.0001	0
PROSB	1	0.188	0.067	2.78	0.0056	0.11037
CONSB	1	-0.326	0.071	-4.55	<0.0001	-0.19888
CONSEFFB	1	0.447	0.054	8.28	<0.0001	0.37322
PSYSXB	1	-0.484	0.072	-6.70	<0.0001	-0.26299

TABLE 4.6
Step 1 of Macro-Level Hierarchical MR Output

Model 1: IVS = PROSB & CONSB, DV = STAGEB

Analysis of Variance

Source	df	Sum of Squares	Mean Square	F-Value	Prob. > F
Model	2	145.72636	72.86318	44.50	<0.0001
Error	524	857.89414	1.63720		
Corrected total	526	1003.62049			
Root MSE		1.27953	*R*-Square	0.1452	
Dep. Mean		2.43643	Adjusted R^2	0.1419	
Coeff Var		52.51662			

and 4.2, we could write the prediction equation for this example as: $Y = A + B1(PROSB) + B2(CONSB) + B3(CONSEFFB) + B4(PSYSXB) + E$. Inserting the unstandardized parameter estimate values from Table 4.5, we have the prediction equation: $Y = 2.705 + 0.188(PROSB) - 0.326(CONSB) + 0.447 (CONSEFFB) - 0.484(PSYSXB) + E$.

Examining the standardized estimates, the strongest predictor of STAGEB is self-efficacy for condom use (i.e., CONSEFFB), which has a standardized beta weight of 0.37. The variable PROSB (i.e., perceptions of the advantages of condom use) is least related to stage of readiness, with a beta weight of 0.11.

Hierarchical Multiple Regression (DV: STAGEB)

With hierarchical MR, the two decisional balance variables, PROSB and CONSB, were entered in the first step (model) based on previous theory (Prochaska et al., 1994a). These two variables were significantly related to STAGEB [$F(2,524) = 44.50$. $p < 0.0001$]. There was a medium multivariate effect size, with $R^2 = 0.15$ and an adjusted R^2 of 0.14. The standardized beta weights for both PROSB ($\beta = 0.22$) and CONSB ($\beta = -0.28$) were slightly larger than when these variables were included with the full set of predictors in the standard MR. See Tables 4.6 and 4.7 for macro- and micro-level output, respectively.

At the second step, Model 2, CONSEFFB has a squared partial correlation of $0.2247 - 0.1452 = 0.0795$, which represents a medium univariate effect size (i.e., >0.06) at that step in the equation. As with the standard MR, and the first step of the hierarchical MR, each of the predictors significantly correlates with STAGEB as indicated by relatively large t-values and small p-values. The standardized beta weights are slightly different than in the first step and in the standard MR, as would be expected with partial coefficients that change depending on other variables in the equation. See Tables 4.8 and 4.9.

TABLE 4.7
Step 1 of Micro-Level Hierarchical MR Output

		Parameter Estimates				
Variable	df	Parameter Estimate	Standard Error	t-value	Prob. > |t|	Standardized Estimate
Intercept	1	1.86865	0.34199	5.46	<.0001	0
PROSB	1	0.37026	0.07016	5.28	<0.0001	0.21629
CONSB	1	−0.45772	0.06719	−6.81	<0.0001	−0.27920

TABLE 4.8
Step 2 of Macro-Level Hierarchical MR Output

Model 2: IVS = PROSB, CONSB, & CONSEFFB, DV = STAGEB

		Analysis of Variance			
Source	df	Sum of Squares	Mean Square	F-Value	Prob. > F
Model	3	225.478	75.159	50.52	<0.0001
Error	523	778.142	1.487		
Corrected total	526	1003.620			
Root MSE		1.21977	R-Square	0.2247	
Dep. Mean		2.43643	Adjusted R^2	0.2202	
Coeff Var		50.06385			

At the final step, Model 3, the variable PSYSXB is added so that at this point there are the full set of four predictors in the equation. Not surprisingly, the statistics look the same as those from the standard MR on these same variables. This shows that the order of entry into the equation makes a difference only during the interim steps when there are varying numbers of variables included. When all variables have been entered, the significance tests (i.e., F and t), effect sizes (e.g., R^2), and

TABLE 4.9
Step 2 of Micro-Level Hierarchical MR Output

		Parameter Estimates				
Variable	df	Parameter Estimate	Standard Error	t-value	Prob. > |t|	Standardized Estimate
Intercept	1	0.60402	0.36895	1.64	0.1022	0
PROSB	1	0.20254	0.07069	2.87	0.0043	0.11832
CONSB	1	−0.21082	0.07239	−2.91	0.0037	−0.12859
CONSEFFB	1	0.40995	0.05599	7.32	<.0001	0.34168

TABLE 4.10
Step 3 of Macro-Level Hierarchical MR Output

Model 3: IVS = PROSB, CONSB, CONSEFFB & PSYSXB, DV = STAGEB

Analysis of Variance

Source	df	Sum of Squares	Mean Square	F-Value	Prob. > F
Model	4	287.06811	71.767	52.28	<0.0001
Error	522	716.55238	1.372		
Corrected total	526	1003.62049			
Root MSE		1.17163	R-Square	0.2860	
Dep. Mean		2.43643	Adjusted R^2	0.2806	
Coeff Var		48.08773			

parameter estimates (i.e., B and β) are the same regardless of their ordering. See Tables 4.10 and 4.11.

Stepwise Multiple Regression (DV: STAGEB)

The stepwise analysis adds variables depending on the magnitude of the correlations among the IVs and outcome variable. Examining the correlation matrix in Table 4.3, we see that the IV with the strongest correlation with STAGEB is CONSEFFB (i.e., $r = 0.447$). Thus, the computer selects this variable to enter first. Though the standardized beta weights are not provided, we can take the square root of the squared semipartial correlation (i.e., $\sqrt{0.2001} = 0.447$) and verify that it is the same as the original correlation because there is only one predictor. See Tables 4.12 and 4.13 for results at the first step.

At Step 2, PSYSXB is added to the equation along with CONSEFFB. This is somewhat surprising given that PSYSXB has the lowest correlation (i.e., -0.10) with STAGEB compared with the other predictors. Based on only the correlations between the IVs and STAGEB, CONSB (i.e., $r = -0.32$ with STAGEB) would

TABLE 4.11
Step 3 of Micro-Level Hierarchical MR Output

Parameter Estimates

Variable	df	Parameter Estimate	Standard Error	t-value	Prob. > |t|	Standardized Estimate
Intercept	1	2.705	0.47328	5.72	<0.0001	0
PROSB	1	0.188	0.06793	2.78	0.0056	0.11037
CONSB	1	−0.326	0.07163	−4.55	<0.0001	−0.19888
CONSEFFB	1	0.44778	0.05408	8.28	<0.0001	0.37322
PSYSXB	1	−0.48491	0.07239	−6.70	<0.0001	−0.26299

TABLE 4.12
Step 1 of Macro-Level Stepwise MR Output

The STEPWISE Procedure MODEL1 Dependent Variable: STAGEB
Forward Selection: Step 1 Variable CONSEFFB Entered:
R-Square = 0.2001

| | | | *Analysis of Variance* | | |
Source	df	Sum of Squares	Mean Square	F-Value	Prob. > F
Model	1	200.869	200.869	131.37	<0.0001
Error	525	802.751	1.529		
Corrected total	526	1003.620			

TABLE 4.13
Step 1 of Micro-Level Stepwise MR Output

| | | | *Parameter Estimates* | | |
Variable	Parameter Estimate	Standard Error	Type II SS	F-Value	Pr > F
Intercept	0.55014	0.17317	15.43298	10.09	0.0016
CONSEFFB	0.53676	0.04683	200.86905	131.37	<0.0001

seem like a reasonable choice for adding at Step 2. However, a glance at the correlations among the IVs reveals that CONSB is moderately correlated (i.e., $r = -0.49$) with CONSEFFB, the variable that entered first. The other IV, PROSB, also has a somewhat moderate correlation (i.e., $r = 0.36$) with CONSEFFB, though PSYSXB does not have much overlap with CONSEFFB (i.e., $r = 0.24$). Thus, the computer selects PSYSXB to enter second into the Stepwise MR equation. Tables 4.14 and 4.15 show results for the second step.

Tables 4.16 and 4.17 present results at Step 3 when CONSB is added to the stepwise regression analysis. Results for Step 4 are given in Tables 4.18 and 4.19, when the final variable, PROSB, is added.

TABLE 4.14
Step 2 of Macro-Level Stepwise MR Output

Stepwise MR (Continued) Forward Selection: Step 2
Variable PSYSXB Entered: R-Square = 0.2472

| | | | *Analysis of Variance* | | |
Source	df	Sum of Squares	Mean Square	F-Value	Prob. > F
Model	2	248.06169	124.03084	86.02	<0.0001
Error	524	755.55881	1.44191		
Corrected total	526	1003.62049			

TABLE 4.15
Step 2 of Micro-Level Stepwise MR Output

| | Parameter Estimates | | | | |
Variable	Parameter Estimate	Standard Error	Type II SS	F-Value	Pr > F
Intercept	1.97403	0.30037	62.27667	43.19	<0.0001
CONSEFFB	0.60101	0.04684	237.36234	164.62	<0.0001
PSYSXB	−0.41184	0.07199	47.19264	32.73	<0.0001

TABLE 4.16
Step 3 of Macro-Level Stepwise MR Output

Stepwise MR (Continued) Forward Selection: Step 3
Variable CONSB Entered: R-Square = 0.2755

| | | | Analysis of Variance | | |
Source	df	Sum of Squares	Mean Square	F-Value	Prob. > F
Model	3	276.45046	92.150	66.28	<0.0001
Error	523	727.17003	1.390		
Corrected total	526	1003.62049			

TABLE 4.17
Step 3 of Micro-Level Stepwise MR Output

| | Parameter Estimates | | | | |
Variable	Parameter Estimate	Standard Error	Type II SS	F-Value	Pr > F
Intercept	3.32566	0.42009	87.13800	62.67	<0.0001
CONSB	−0.32572	0.07208	28.38877	20.42	<0.0001
CONSEFFB	0.49670	0.05147	129.50105	93.14	<0.0001
PSYSXB	−0.49093	0.07283	63.18512	45.44	<0.0001

TABLE 4.18
Step 4 of Macro-Level Stepwise MR Output

Stepwise MR (Continued) Forward Selection: Step 4
Variable PROSB Entered: R-Square = 0.2860

| | | | Analysis of Variance | | |
Source	df	Sum of Squares	Mean Square	F-Value	Prob. > F
Model	4	287.06811	71.767	52.28	<0.0001
Error	522	716.55238	1.372		
Corrected total	526	1003.62049			

TABLE 4.19
Step 4 of Micro-Level Stepwise MR Output

Variable	Parameter Estimates				
	Parameter Estimate	Standard Error	Type II SS	F-Value	Pr > F
Intercept	2.70524	0.47328	44.84867	32.67	<0.0001
PROSB	0.18893	0.06793	10.61765	7.73	0.0056
CONSB	−0.32605	0.07163	28.44600	20.72	<0.0001
CONSEFFB	0.44778	0.05408	94.11412	68.56	<0.0001
PSYSXB	−0.48491	0.07239	61.58991	44.87	<0.0001

Note in Table 4.19 that this final stepwise model is the same as the last step in hierarchical and standard MR, because all the variables were included in the equation for each MR. If only a subset of variables were significant in the stepwise MR, the final equation would have fewer variables than in hierarchical and standard MR and the final output would not be the same for stepwise MR. In each form of MR (standard, hierarchical, and stepwise), all four predictor variables were entered into the model, providing the same results for the final output.

Table 4.20 provides a summary of the four steps in the stepwise MR for this example with R-Squares, F-Values, and probability values for each step.

Notice that in all three forms of MR (standard, hierarchical, and stepwise), the contribution of PSYSXB seems to be larger in the presence of other variables than the simple correlation between PSYSXB and STAGEB (i.e., $r = -0.10$). This suggests that PSYSXB may be what is called a suppressor variable that facilitates relationships within an analysis. Though discussion of this kind of variable is beyond the scope of this book, interested readers are encouraged to examine this in more detail elsewhere (Cohen, Cohen, West, & Aiken, 2003; Tabachnick & Fidell, 2001; Grimm & Yarnold, 1995).

Figure 4.2 depicts the four predictors of stage of condom use, with the standardized coefficients found from the final step in standard, hierarchical, and stepwise

TABLE 4.20
Summary of Micro-Level Stepwise MR Output

	Summary of Forward Selection			
Step	1	2	3	4
Variable Entered	CONSEFFB	PSYSXB	CONSB	PROSB
Number of Variables in	1	2	3	4
Partial R-Square	0.2001	0.0470	0.0283	0.0106
Model R-Square	0.2001	0.2472	0.2755	0.2860
Adjusted R-Square	0.1940	0.2414	0.2700	0.2805
F-Value	131.3700	32.7300	20.4200	7.7300
Pr > F	<0.0001	<0.0001	<0.0001	0.0056

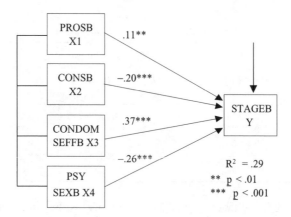

FIG. 4.2. MR with 4 xs and 1 Y showing significant R^2 shared variance, $F(4,522)=52.28$, $p < 0.001$, and significant standardized regression coefficients. Lines connecting the three IVs depict correlations among predictors and the arrow headed toward the outcome variable represents prediction error.

TABLE 4.21

Multiplicity, Background, Central, and Interpretation Themes Applied to Multiple Regression

Themes	Multiple Regression
Multiplicity themes (Note: + means multiplicity of theme pertains)	+*Theory, Hypotheses & Empirical Research* +*Controls*: Covariate(s) of Confound(s) added +*Time Points*: IVs &/or DV +*Samples*: Cross-validate +*Measurements*: +IVs, 1 DV, +Covariates
Background themes	*Sample Data*: Random selection, large (5–50): N/p ratio *Measures*: Continuous IVs & covariate(s), continuous DV *Assumptions*: Normality, linearity, homoscedasticity *Methods*: Inferential with random data and assumptions met
Central themes	$X' =$ *linear combination of X variables (relate this to Y)* *Variance*: in DV (both explained: R^2, and unexplained: $1 - R^2$) *Covariance*: between DV and IVs and among IVs *Ratio*: R^2 explained variance/$(1 - R^2)$ unexplained variance
Interpretation themes and Questions to Ask	*Macro*: F-test, effect size *Micro*: t-tests, regression weights Do IVs significantly predict or relate to DV? Are all variables reliable and needed? Low correlations among IVs (i.e., no collinearity)? Significant R^2 or shared variance between IVs and DV? Significant subset(s) of IVs? Which IVs significantly predict DV? Assumptions met? Have possible confounds been considered?

MR analyses conducted on these data. Though it is not always the case, the results were the same because all variables were retained in all three analyses. For ease of presentation, values for the correlations among the predictor variables and prediction error are not indicated in Figure 4.2.

These results suggested that almost 30% of the variance in stage of condom use is associated with the four predictors. Beginning with variables that contributed the most, with standardized regression coefficients (β) given in parentheses, stage of condom use is associated with greater perceived self-efficacy for using condoms ($\beta = 0.37$), less positive psychosexual functioning ($\beta = -0.26$), less perceived disadvantages (i.e., cons) of condom use ($\beta = -0.20$), and greater perceived advantages (i.e., pros) of condom use ($\beta = 0.11$). Ideally, these results should be replicated in a larger, more diverse, and random sample.

SUMMARY

Table 4.21 summarizes how the main multiplicity, background, central, and interpretation themes apply to MR.

REFERENCES

Cohen, J. (1988). *Statistical power analysis for the behavioral sciences.* San Diego, CA: Academic Press.

Cohen, J. (1992). A power primer. *Psychological Bulletin, 112,* 155–159.

Cohen, J., Cohen, P., West, S.G., & Aiken, L.S. (2003). *Applied multiple regression/correlation analysis for behavioral sciences* (3rd ed.). Mahwah, NJ: Lawrence Erlbaum Associates.

Goldman, J. A., & Harlow, L. L. (1993). Self-perception variables that mediate AIDS preventive behavior in college students. *Health Psychology, 12,* 489–498.

Green, S. B. (1991). How many subjects does it take to do a regression analysis? *Multivariate Behavioral Research, 26,* 449–510.

Grimm, L. G., & Yarnold, P. R. (1995). *Reading and understanding multivariate statistics* (Ch. 2, pp. 19–64). Washington, DC: APA.

Harlow, L. L., Quina, K., Morokoff, P. J., Rose, J. S., & Grimley, D. (1993). HIV risk in women: A multifaceted model. *Journal of Applied Biobehavioral Research, 1,* 3–38.

Harlow, L., Rose, J., Morokoff, P., Quina, K., Mayer, K., Mitchell, K. & Schnoll, R. (1998). Women HIV sexual risk takers: Related behaviors, interpersonal issues & attitudes. *Women's Health: Research on Gender, Behavior and Policy, 4,* 407–439.

Kirk, R. E. (1996). Practical significance: A concept whose time has come. *Educational and Psychological Measurement, 56,* 746–759.

Marcus, B. H., Eaton, C. A., Rossi, J. S., & Harlow, L. L. (1994). Self-efficacy, decision-making and stages of change: A model of physical exercise. *Journal of Applied Social Psychology, 24,* 489–508.

Pedhazur, E. J. (1997). *Multiple regression in behavioral research: Explanation and prediction* (3rd ed.). Fort Worth, TX: Harcourt Brace College Publishers.

Prochaska, J. O., Redding, C. A., Harlow, L. L., Rossi, J. S., & Velicer, W. F. (1994a). The Transtheoretical model and HIV prevention: A review. *Health Education Quarterly, 21,* 45–60.

Prochaska, J. O., Velicer, W. F., Rossi, J. S., Goldstein, M. G., Marcus, B. H., Rakowski, W., Fiore, C., Harlow, L. L., Redding, C. A., Rosenbloom, D., & Rossi, S. R. (1994b). Stages of change and decisional balance for 12 problem behaviors. *Health Psychology, 13*, 39–46.

Prochaska, J. O., & Velicer, W. F. (1997). The transtheoretical model of health behavior change. *American Journal of Health Promotion, 12*, 38–48.

SAS (1999). *Statistical Analysis Software, Release 8.1.* Cary, NC: SAS Institute Inc.

Tabachnick, B. G., & Fidell, L. S. (2001). *Using multivariate statistics* (4th ed.: Ch. 5, pp. 111–176). Boston: Allyn and Bacon.

5

Analysis of Covariance

Themes Applied to Analysis of Covariance (ANCOVA)

Similar to multiple regression (MR), ANCOVA can be viewed as an intermediate method. The features and uses for ANCOVA help form a useful transition from univariate/bivariate methods such as analysis of variance (ANOVA) and MR to more rigorous multivariate methods such as multivariate analysis of variance (MANOVA) and canonical correlation, among others. As with MR, it is instructive to view ANCOVA through the lens of various kinds of themes. We will approach ANCOVA with the same 10 questions used with MR and see where it takes us.

WHAT IS ANCOVA AND HOW IS IT SIMILAR TO AND DIFFERENT FROM OTHER METHODS?

ANCOVA allows us to assess whether there are significant group differences on a single continuous dependent variable (DV), after controlling for the effects of one or more continuous independent variables (IVs), called covariates. ANCOVA allows one or more categorical IVs and one continuous DV, *plus* one or more co-variates. Thus, ANCOVA always has at least two IVs (i.e., one or more categorical, grouping IVs, and one or more continuous covariates).

ANCOVA can be viewed as a combination of ANOVA and MR in that the focus is on separating groups as well as correlating variables. In the ANOVA portion, we try to select variables that will show as much separation as possible between the groups of the IV on the single continuous DV. In the MR portion, we focus on identifying continuous variables that relate strongly to the DV but that are not highly interrelated on the IV side. In this way, ANCOVA can be thought of as a type of partial correlation analysis, where the focus is on the relationship between the IVs and the DV with the effect of the covariate(s) partialed out of the DV.

ANCOVA requires the following pattern of correlations:

a. **Covariates should be at least moderately correlated with the DV** (e.g., $r > 0.30$). This makes it worthwhile to use up an extra degree of freedom for each covariate that is included. If the correlation between a covariate and a DV is too small, very little variance will be partialed out of the DV before examining group differences. At the same time, the degrees of freedom for the error term are reduced, although the actual error term itself is not reduced substantially, leading to a slightly higher critical value that is required to reach significance than would be the case without adding the covariate. Thus, the calculated F-test has to jump a little higher when covariates are added. If the covariate is substantially correlated with the DV, the loss in a degree of freedom is more than compensated by the reduction in error variance, making it easier to reach significance.

b. **Covariates should be reliably measured** (e.g., reliability coefficient >0.70). Correlations between unreliable variables are less powerful than those with high reliability. As we just saw in the previous suggestion, covariates that are not highly correlated with the DV are less apt to contribute to an analysis.

c. **There should be low correlations among covariates** if multiple continuous variables are added to an ANCOVA design. Variables that are highly correlated within a side (e.g., within IVs) lead to collinearity problems (e.g., instability and bias). Thus, it is always best to choose covariates that are relatively uncorrelated with each other.

d. **Similarly, there should not be any appreciable correlation between covariates and grouping variables**. In addition to collinearity problems, this could lead to a violation of an important assumption in ANCOVA, that of homogeneity of regressions. We will discuss this assumption more later. For now, consider that, when a covariate is inadvertently correlated with a grouping variable at the same time that it is correctly correlated with the DV, the relationship between the covariate and the DV will be different depending on the group to which a participant is assigned. For much the same reason that we need homogeneity of variance assumptions (i.e., equal variances across groups) to pool results across groups, we also need to have a similar relationship between a covariate and a DV at each level of the IV. Thus, significant correlation between a covariate and a grouping IV can lead to violation of the assumption of homogeneity of regression, thereby invalidating the use of ANCOVA.

ANCOVA is similar to and an extension of ANOVA in that they both examine group differences with the same kinds of IVs and DV. ANCOVA, however, has greater capability to fine-tune the nature of the group differences by including other possible confounding IVs or covariates. In essence, we are examining how much groups differ on a DV that is separate from any relationships with other extraneous variables. In this way, we get a purer picture of group differences than when just using ANOVA that does not allow the use of any covariates. ANCOVA can also be seen as somewhat similar to MR in that they both have multiple IVs and a single DV. ANCOVA differs from MR in that we always have both categorical and continuous IVs with ANCOVA. Interested readers can investigate other discussions of ANCOVA (Hair, Anderson, Tatham, & Black, 2004; Pedhazur, 1997; Rutherford, 2001; Tabachnick & Fidell, 2001).

WHEN IS ANCOVA USED AND WHAT RESEARCH QUESTIONS CAN IT ADDRESS?

There are three main uses for ANCOVA, the last of which is somewhat controversial:

a. **Experimental Design.** ANCOVA can be used in an experimental design, to control for initial levels of some continuous variable(s) (e.g., pretest scores on the DV). With this design, the categorical grouping variable would be manipulated and participants would be randomly assigned to different groups, at least one of which is a treatment condition. For example, we could examine differences in smoking levels for three treatment programs for quitting smoking, after partialing (i.e., covarying) out initial levels of smoking and other possible confounding variables (e.g., stress, number of individuals smoking in a participant's environment). This would provide a sensitive test of the veracity of the treatment programs that took into account other factors that could affect participants' smoking levels on top of the experimental treatment condition. ANCOVA is always preferable to ANOVA when we think background or confounding variables also might be related to the DV, over and above the manipulated IV.

b. **Stringent follow-up to MANOVA.** ANCOVAs can be used as follow-ups to a significant MANOVA, where each DV in MANOVA is successively used as the single DV in ANCOVA, with other DVs held as covariates. For example, we could examine which DV is showing significant differences among three treatment groups on two DVs, by running an ANCOVA on each of the DVs separately, where the other DV serves as a covariate. This would provide a stringent test of group differences on a DV over and above any differences on other DVs (see more in Chapter 7).

c. **Non- or quasi-experimental design.** ANCOVA has also been used to statistically control for differences in one or more variables in a non- or quasi-experimental design with intact groups. This use is controversial and not always recommended because it is nearly impossible to consider all possible covariates that could be relevant to the study. In this type of design, we do not have the luxury of randomly assigning participants to treatments, which essentially would control for all possible confounds. Instead, we have to scour the literature and our own thinking to consider what other variables should be included to get a clear test of potential differences between intact groups on a single outcome variable. One of the more famous uses of quasi-experimental ANCOVA concerns evaluation of the Head Start program. Briefly, two intact groups were compared: Young children who came from disadvantaged backgrounds and those from more privileged backgrounds. Youngsters who were disadvantaged were offered a Head Start treatment that was expected to help enrich their learning experience and improve school performance. To get a fair assessment of any differences between the two groups, relevant covariates had to be taken into account (e.g., family income, parents' education) that were believed also to relate to school performance. One of the problems with this use of ANCOVA is that there is no way of considering all possible confounds, and thus the statistical control is often faulty or misleading. Still, it is sometimes worthwhile to use this form of ANCOVA, keeping in mind the limitations in the conclusions made. We certainly would not have the option of making causal statements about the effects of the treatment because there could be dozens of other factors that could have affected the DV, over and above that of the quasi- or nonexperimental IV.

WHAT ARE THE MAIN MULTIPLICITY THEMES FOR ANCOVA?

ANCOVA offers several ways to consider the theme of multiplicity. As with MR, it is instructive and even essential that multiple theories and empirical studies be investigated before conducting an ANCOVA. These hopefully would yield avenues to approach a design to offer the best opportunities for articulating rigorous hypotheses with which to draw clear inferences from the data. A categorical, possibly treatment-based, IV would need to be selected, along with a pertinent, continuous DV. Of course, one or more reliable covariates should emerge that would help to statistically isolate the relationship between the IV and the DV. Ideally, one or more random samples would be identified in which participants could be randomly assigned to one of the manipulated groups of the IV. If possible, data could be collected over two or more time points, with initial measures used as covariates and a follow-up measure used as the DV. This would allow an examination of whether there were significant differences on a DV after statistically controlling for the initial levels of that variable. If the design is experimental, there is greater capability of making causal conclusions about the effects of the IV. With non- or quasi-experimental designs, it still may be useful to consider ANCOVA, especially when including multiple covariates that would help in ruling out extraneous confounds and build in some control over findings, although certainly not as much as when using a large, random sample in an experimental design.

WHAT ARE THE MAIN BACKGROUND THEMES APPLIED TO ANCOVA?

Just as we did with MR, we should consider what background themes should be addressed for ANCOVA. Certainly it would be helpful to have a large ($N \times p$) data matrix that included at least one categorical, grouping IV, a single, continuous DV, and one or more continuous covariates. It is important to recognize that every covariate will use up one degree of freedom (df) so that it will become harder to reject the null hypothesis of no group differences with many covariates. If a covariate is reliable and pertinent to the study (e.g., strongly relates to the DV and has little or no relationship with the IV), then the power of the study is increased, making it worth the loss of df. However, if too many, possibly irrelevant covariates are added, the power of the study could weaken, making it very difficult to find any effects that might truly be present. Another consideration is the nature of the sample. Whenever possible it is best to maintain approximately equal numbers of participants for each group because this makes the analysis more robust. It is also worthwhile to conduct a power analysis (Cohen, 1988) to determine the number of participants needed per group to allow the greatest chance of finding the expected effect.

Descriptive statistics should always be conducted to examine means and standard deviations across groups. Reliability coefficients should be calculated for all variables, particularly the covariates. As with MR, the continuous IVs (called covariates in ANCOVA) are assumed to be measured without error and to be perfectly reliable. Although this is very difficult to ensure in practice, every effort should be made to obtain reliable measures.

To allow for inferences beyond a specific study, assumptions should hold. These include the same three mentioned for MR— namely normality, linearity, and homoscedasticity. An examination of skewness, kurtosis, and bivariate scatter plots can help verify the latter assumptions. Another assumption, unique to ANCOVA, is the assumption of homogeneity of regressions. This assumption requires that the regression coefficient between the covariate and DV is the same at each level of the IV. Some think this assumption requires that the means on the covariate be the same at each level of the IV. This is not what is addressed with this assumption, though certainly it would be helpful to have all groups equal before starting a study. Because ANCOVA takes covariates into account in the ANOVA between the IV(s) and DV, it is important that the degree of relationship between the covariate(s) and DV be similar across groups so that the statistical correction is evenly made for each group.

With a sufficient-sized sample that is randomly drawn from a relevant population, random assignment of participants to manipulated groups, reliable and well-chosen variables, and a reasonable degree of met assumptions, inferences may be generalized to the larger population of interest. Of course, meeting all these ideals is very difficult to accomplish in most research studies. The best advice is to proceed with caution using the best design that resources allow.

WHAT IS THE STATISTICAL MODEL THAT IS TESTED WITH ANCOVA?

The theoretical model of ANCOVA is similar to the model for ANOVA. The ANOVA model can be written as:

$$Y = \mu_y + \tau + E, \tag{5.1}$$

where Y is a continuous outcome variable, μ_y is the grand mean of all Y scores across all groups of the IV(s), τ is a treatment effect, and E indicates error.

The ANCOVA model adds the weighted effect of the covariate(s):

$$Y = \mu_y + \tau + [B_i(C_i - M_{ci}) + \cdots] + E, \tag{5.2}$$

where B_i represents an unstandardized regression coefficient (similar to that for MR) corresponding to the ith covariate, C_i, M_{ci} is the mean of the ith covariate, and E is error variance.

The similarity with and difference between the ANOVA and ANCOVA models can be seen even more readily by noting that ANCOVA is simply an ANOVA on Y scores that have been adjusted for the effects of the covariates, C:

$$Y - [B_i(C_i - M_{xi}) + \cdots] = \mu_y + \tau + E \tag{5.3}$$

Equation 5.3 shows that, when the DV is adjusted for the effects of the covariate, this adjusted Y-score can be modeled just like the unadjusted Y in the ANOVA model (though we use up an extra df for each covariate that is added). Thus, ANCOVA can be viewed as an ANOVA on Y scores in which the relationships between the covariates and the DV are partialed out of the DV.

Similar to what is done with MR, we examine a regression line between two continuous variables. Whereas in MR the regression is between an IV and the DV, in ANCOVA the regression is between a covariate, C, and the DV. Of course a covariate *is* an IV, much like an IV in MR, though it is not usually the main focus in an ANCOVA where one or more categorical IVs are often examined as the main focus for explaining the variance in an outcome variable, Y. Another distinction is that in MR we think of adding extra continuous variables to improve prediction, whereas we often add continuous covariates in ANCOVA to reduce the within-groups error term. Thus, in ANCOVA, we often think of identifying and partialing out unwanted variance that otherwise would be delegated to the within-groups error variance. When the error term (used in the denominator of an F-test) is smaller, the overall F-ratio generally will be larger with ANCOVA making it easier to reach macro-level significance.

HOW DO CENTRAL THEMES OF VARIANCE, COVARIANCE, AND LINEAR COMBINATIONS APPLY TO ANCOVA?

Just as with ANOVA, in ANCOVA we are very interested in the ratio of between-groups variance over within-groups variance. To reject a hypothesis that there are no significant differences across groups, we would expect that the variance between the group means on the DV would be substantially larger than the average variance of the DV within each of the groups. We also would like to see a significant covariance between the covariate and the DV, thereby allowing us to subtract this systematic variance from the error term. The linear combination that is examined in ANCOVA is the Y score that is adjusted for the effects of the covariates (see Equation 5.3 above). Just as MR allows an examination of shared variance between the IV(s) and DV (i.e., R^2), in ANCOVA we can examine the proportion of shared variance between the adjusted Y score and the IV(s). In ANCOVA, as with ANOVA, this is often referred to as Eta-squared (i.e., η^2), which is a ratio of the sum of squares (i.e., numerator of a variance term or the sum of squared differences between a score and a mean) due to a specific effect (e.g., between groups or interaction effect), over the total sum of squares:

$$\eta^2 = (SS_{\text{effect}})/(SS_{\text{total}}) \tag{5.4}$$

Like R^2, η^2 is a proportion ranging from 0 to 1. We will find out more about η^2 in the next section, which examines macro-level interpretation of ANCOVA results.

WHAT ARE THE MAIN THEMES NEEDED TO INTERPRET ANCOVA RESULTS AT A MACRO-LEVEL?

When conducting ANCOVA, it is important to evaluate results at the omnibus or macro-level before examining more specific, micro-level aspects. Macro-level assessment for ANCOVA involves a significance test and an effect size. η^2 is often calculated to get an effect size or percentage of variance in the DV that is explained by the IVs.

Significance Test

As with ANOVA and MR, the main overall index of fit in ANCOVA is the F-test. If the F-test is significant in ANCOVA (e.g., $p < 0.05$), we can conclude that there are significant mean differences between at least two groups, after taking into account one or more covariates.

Effect Size (ES)

In ANCOVA, as with ANOVA, we would like to examine the magnitude of the relationship between the IV(s) and the DV. This can be done with η^2, which was just described as the ratio of the sum of squares for an effect over the total sum of squares (SS), where both SS are adjusted for the effects of the covariates. As with R^2, we can interpret η^2 values for ANCOVA with multivariate guidelines for a small effect size when equal to about 0.02, a medium effect size when equal to about 0.13, and a large effect size when greater than or equal to about 0.26. I have also seen researchers adopt univariate guidelines for ES with ANCOVA, especially when using only one grouping IV and one covariate. It is probably best to leave the choice up to the researcher depending on whether a more conservative approach is needed (calling for the larger multivariate ESs) in a well-known area of research, or a more statistically powerful approach (using 0.01, 0.06, and 0.13 univariate ESs) when conducting an exploratory study in an area that is not well researched.

WHAT ARE THE MAIN THEMES
NEEDED TO INTERPRET ANCOVA
RESULTS AT A MICRO-LEVEL?

If the macro-level F-test is significant in ANCOVA, we can then feel free to examine where the significance lies. Just as with ANOVA, this most likely involves significance tests of specific group differences and effect sizes for group means.

a. **Follow-up planned comparisons** (e.g., post hoc, simple effects, etc.) provide a specific examination of which groups are showing differences. Tukey (1953) tests of an honestly significant difference (HSD) between a pair of means provide some protection for overall error rate. Though I tend to conduct Tukey tests using a stringent alpha level of 0.01, this may be too conservative. As with the choice of ES guidelines, I leave the selection of a p-value size to the researcher's good judgment, something we have to rely on more often than we would like to think in science.

b. **Cohen's *d* can provide an ES** for the difference between a pair of means (Cohen, 1988, 1992). This is easily calculated as:

$$d = (M_1 - M_2)/\text{pooled standard deviation} \qquad (5.5)$$

where d is the standardized difference between means, M_i is the mean of group i, and the denominator in Equation 5.5 is the average standard deviation of Y across all the IV groups. A value of 0.20 for Cohen's (1988) d is interpreted as a small ES, a value of 0.50 represents a medium ES, and a value of 0.80 or larger indicates a large ES.

c. **Graphs of means** for each group also provide a qualitative examination of specific differences between groups. Plotting the mean values for Y along a vertical axis and plotting the various groups for the IV along a horizontal axis easily accomplish this. Visual trends can be examined by noting the pattern of the means. If a horizontal line can be drawn to link the mean values between groups, the means are not different. If a line drawn between the group means is sloped, there is some evidence that the group means differ.

WHAT ARE SOME OTHER CONSIDERATIONS OR NEXT STEPS AFTER APPLYING ANCOVA?

After conducting an ANCOVA, it would be useful to evaluate how well the design could support causal inferences as well as generalizations beyond the immediate sample. Both of these considerations would be strengthened if an experimental design were implemented on a large and random sample, with random assignment to groups. Results should be replicated on an independent sample and variables should be carefully reevaluated as to their appropriateness and reliability for use in ANCOVA. If a covariate does not seem to be sufficiently related to the DV of interest, or if it is demonstrating some correlation with a grouping IV (resulting in heterogeneity of regression), then other more well-behaved covariates should be considered for future study. To the extent that selected covariates worked well in ANCOVA conducted within an experimental design, control of background variables can be reasonably achieved allowing for some isolation of the main effects and possible causal interpretation.

WHAT IS AN EXAMPLE OF APPLYING ANCOVA TO A RESEARCH QUESTION?

Here is an example of ANCOVA where the initial time 1 ($t1$) Stage (STAGEA) of condom use is the IV (with 5 ordinal levels: 1, precontemplation; 2, contemplation;

3, preparation; 4, action; and 5, maintenance), the cons of condom use at $t1$ (CONSA) serve as the covariate, and the cons of condom use at $t2$, 6 months later (CONSB) serve as the DV. With respect to multiplicity, we can note that the continuous variable, cons, is measured over multiple time points and that there are multiple IVs (i.e., the categorical IV of STAGEA, and the continuous covariate IV of CONSA), though little else about the design draws on the theme of multiplicity. Both measures of the cons of condom use are average scores of 5 or 6 quasi-continuous items assessed on a 5-point Likert scale. Items list several reasons why someone might not use a condom (e.g., "sex is not exciting") and ask how important each reason would be when thinking about whether to use a condom (ranging from 1 = not at all important to 5 = very important). Thus, higher scores for either CONSA or CONSB indicate greater importance attached to a reason not to use condoms.

As with the MR example, this ANCOVA example draws on the theory of the transtheoretical model specifically as it relates to decisional balance and the stages of change (Prochaska et al, 1994). We should realize that our example is one of the more controversial applications of ANCOVA because we use intact groups of participants who naturally fall into one of the five stages of condom use. Thus, we present an application that should be interpreted cautiously at a descriptive rather than an inferential level.

Remember that throughout these and other analyses, variables from the initial time point are labeled with "A" at the end, whereas variables measured 6 months later have "B" at the end. Because the IV: STAGEA, and covariate: CONSA, are measured at the initial time point, whereas the DV: CONSB, is measured 6 months later, we can assess whether individuals at the varying stages of condom use differ on their perceived disadvantages to condom use, after controlling for or taking into account initial perceptions of the disadvantages to condom use, 6 months earlier.

Analyses are conducted with the SAS (1999) computer program. For all macro-level significance tests (i.e., ANOVA and ANCOVA F-tests), the alpha level is set at a conventional $p < 0.05$. For micro-level analyses (e.g., Tukey tests), I adopt a more stringent alpha level of $p < 0.01$ to provide some protection for Type I error rate. If a major goal were to decrease Type II errors (i.e., protect against holding on to the null hypothesis when it should be rejected), it would be reasonable to consider an alpha level of 0.05 that would provide greater power. Output is provided and discussed for several sets of analyses: A, descriptive statistics; B, correlations; C, test of homogeneity of regressions; D, ANOVA; and E, ANCOVA.

Descriptive Statistics

Table 5.1 presents descriptive statistics for the variables used in this analysis of covariance example. From the frequencies presented for the IV, STAGEA, we see that there are 527 participants who contributed data for these analyses. Individuals

TABLE 5.1
ANCOVA Example Descriptive Statistics

STAGEA	Frequency	Percent	Cumulative Frequency	Cumulative Percent
1 = Precontemplation	151	28.65	151	28.65
2 = Contemplation	204	38.71	355	67.36
3 = Preparation	70	13.28	425	80.65
4 = Action	20	3.80	445	84.44
5 = Maintenance	82	15.56	527	100.00

Variable	Mean	S.D.	Min.	Max.	Skewness	Kurtosis
STAGEA	2.39	1.35	1.00	5.00	0.89	−0.40
CONSA	2.14	0.90	1.00	5.00	0.71	0.08
CONSB	2.05	0.84	1.00	5.00	0.89	0.49

are unevenly distributed across the five stages of condom use, with most in the contemplation stage where they are considering possible condom use. The next most endorsed category is the precontemplation stage where 151 of the 527 individuals are not even considering the use of condoms. The least endorsed category is the action stage where only 20 individuals (i.e., 4%) report that they have consistently used condoms for the last 6 months or less. Having unequal cell sizes for the five stages is not optimal for ANCOVA, nor is it preferable to have naturally occurring, intact stages where participants are not randomly assigned. Still, the analysis can provide descriptive information on whether perceived disadvantages to using condoms differ after 6 months for individuals at various stages of readiness to use condoms, while controlling for initial perceived cons of condom use.

From the means, standard deviations, skewness, and kurtosis values, it appears that all variables are relatively normally distributed, with low levels of endorsement on the one to five point scales. All three variables exhibit slight skewness (i.e., see values close to 1.0). Still, the means do not reach ceiling or floor levels and are all greater than their standard deviations, suggesting reasonably even distributions for the variables.

Correlations

As shown in Table 5.2, there is a relatively strong correlation ($r = 0.61$) between the covariate (i.e., CONSA) and the DV (CONSB), as is needed. The size of this correlation indicates reasonable test-retest reliability over 6 months on the perceived disadvantages to using condoms. The ordinal variables, STAGEA and STAGEB correlate moderately high (i.e., $r = 0.67$), also suggesting fairly stable test-retest reliability over a 6-month period and relatively static stages of change in this naturalistic study.

TABLE 5.2
Pearson Correlation Coefficients ($N = 527$)

	CONSA	CONSB	STAGEA	STAGEB
		Prob > |r| under H0: Rho = 0		
CONSA	1.000	0.613	−0.300	−0.246
		<0.0001	<0.0001	<0.0001
CONSB	0.613	1.000	0.293	−0.316
	<0.0001		<0.0001	<0.0001
STAGEA	−0.300	−0.293	1.000	0.670
	<0.0001	<0.0001		<0.0001
STAGEB	−0.246	−0.316	0.670	1.000
	<0.0001	<0.0001	<0.0001	

Finally, there is also a relatively small, though not zero, significant correlation (i.e., $r = -0.30$) between the IV (STAGEA) and the covariate (CONSA). Remember that the assumption of homogeneity of regressions assumes that the slopes between the covariate and DV are similar across all levels of the IV. This assumption implies that the covariate and IV are not correlated. Even the relatively small correlation (i.e., $r = -0.30$) found here could lead to possible problems with heterogeneity of regressions when conducting an ANCOVA on these data later on. A possible violation of the assumption of homogeneity of regressions will be examined more closely in the next section.

Test of Homogeneity of Regressions

Note in Table 5.3 that the interaction between the covariate, CONSA, and the IV, STAGEA, is not significant. The lack of significance suggests that the assumption of homogeneity of regressions holds for this analysis, allowing us to proceed with ANCOVA on these data. Before doing so, however, it is helpful to first conduct an ANOVA on these data, allowing a basis for comparing subsequent results from an ANCOVA.

ANOVA and Follow-up Tukey Tests

When a simple one-way ANOVA is conducted on these data, Table 5.4 reveals that it shows a significant macro-effect for STAGEA, $F(4,522) = 12.49$, $p < 0.0001$, $R^2 = \eta^2 = SS_{\text{Effect}}/SS_{\text{Total}} = 0.09$, which represents a medium, univariate effect size or a small to medium multivariate ES (Cohen, 1988, 1992). This suggests that 9% of the variance in the perceived disadvantages to condom use can be explained by an individual's readiness to use condoms 6 months earlier. It is not a very large ES, and we certainly cannot establish a causal link given the nonexperimental data. Still, it is worthwhile to examine micro-results of means and

TABLE 5.3

Testing for Homogeneity of Regressions

The GLM Procedure: Class Level Information

Class	Levels	Values
STAGEA	5	1 2 3 4 5

Number of observations   527
Dependent Variable: CONSB

Source	df	Sum of Squares	Mean Square	F-Value	Prob. > F
Model	9	146.7026427	16.3002936	37.17	<0.0001
Error	517	226.7024807	0.4384961		
Corrected total	526	373.4051233			
Root MSE		0.662190	R-Square	0.392878	
Dependent Mean		2.051550			
Coeff Var		32.27757			

Source	df	Type III SS	Mean Square	F-Value	Prob. > F
CONSA	1	58.96091371	58.96091371	134.46	<0.0001
STAGEA	4	1.01389539	0.25347385	0.58	0.6787
CONSA* STAGEA	4	0.89363979	0.22340995	0.51	0.7288

TABLE 5.4

ANOVA Macro-Level Results

The GLM Procedure: Class Level Information

Class	Levels	Values
STAGEA	5	1 2 3 4 5

Number of observations   527
Dependent Variable: CONSB

Source	df	Sum of Squares	Mean Square	F-Value	Prob. > F
Model	4	32.6189479	8.1547370	12.49	<0.0001
Error	522	340.7861755	0.6528471		
Corrected total	526	373.4051233			
Root MSE		0.807990	R-Square	0.087355	
Dependent Mean		2.051550			
Coeff Var		39.38435			

Source	df	Type III SS	Mean Square	F-Value	Prob. > F
STAGEA	4	32.61894788	8.15473697	12.49	<0.0001

TABLE 5.5
Micro-Level Tukey Tests for ANOVA

The GLM Procedure: Least Squares Means
Adjustment for Multiple Comparisons: Tukey-Kramer

STAGEA	CONSB LSMEAN	99% Confidence	Limits
1 = Precontemplation	2.279249	2.109259	2.449240
2 = Contemplation	2.136438	1.990187	2.282689
3 = Preparation	2.002381	1.752712	2.252050
4 = Action	1.691667	1.224579	2.158754
5 = Maintenance	1.550813	1.320135	1.781491

Least Squares Means for effect STAGEA Pr > |t| for H0:
LSMean(i) = LSMean(j) Dependent Variable: CONSB

i/j	1	2	3	4	5
1		0.4684	0.1253	0.0199	<0.0001
2	0.4684		0.7527	0.1313	<0.0001
3	0.1253	0.7527		0.5520	0.0058
4	0.0199	0.1313	0.5520		0.9567
5	<0.0001	<0.0001	0.0058	0.9567	

Least Squares Means for Effect STAGEA

i	j	Difference Between Means	Simultaneous 99% Confidence Limits for LSMean(i)-LSMean(j)	
1	2	0.142812	−0.140971	0.426594
1	3	0.276868	−0.105369	0.659106
1	4	0.587583	−0.041444	1.216609
1	5	0.728436	0.365812	1.091061*
2	3	0.134057	−0.232115	0.500229
2	4	0.444771	−0.174625	1.064167
2	5	0.585625	0.239976	0.931274*
3	4	0.310714	−0.359528	0.980956
3	5	0.451568	0.021398	0.881738*
4	5	0.140854	−0.518400	0.800107

*Mean differences that are indicated with an asterisk are significant. Thus, STAGE 5 is significantly different from STAGES 1, 2 & 3.

Tukey planned comparison tests to assess whether there are any significant differences in perceived disadvantages to condom use, across the five stages of condom use.

Table 5.5 presents the micro-level Tukey tests for the significant macro-level F-test in the ANOVA just conducted. Notice that there are significant mean differences between STAGE 5, and stages 1, 2, and 3. Thus, individuals in the maintenance stage of condom use (i.e., regularly using a condom for 6 months or longer) report having significantly fewer perceived disadvantages to using condoms than

TABLE 5.6
ANCOVA Macro-Level Results

The GLM Procedure: Class Level Information

Class		Levels	Values
STAGEA		5	1 2 3 4 5

Number of observations   527
Dependent Variable: CONSB

Source	df	Sum of Squares	Mean Square	F-Value	Prob. > F
Model	5	145.8090029	29.1618006	66.76	<0.0001
Error	521	227.5961205	0.4368448		
Corrected total	526	373.4051233			
Root MSE		0.660942	R-Square	0.390485	
Dependent Mean		2.051550			
Coeff Var		32.21674			

Source	df	Type III SS	Mean Square	F-Value	Prob. > F
CONSA	1	113.1900550	113.1900550	259.11	<0.0001
STAGEA	4	5.2795469	1.3198867	3.02	0.0176

individuals in either precontemplation (i.e., never thinking about using condoms), contemplation (i.e., starting to think about using condoms), or preparation (i.e., beginning to take steps to using condoms) stages.

It is now useful to conduct an ANCOVA on these same data that controls for the effects of initial perceived disadvantages of condom use (i.e., CONSA). In an ideal experimental design, where individuals are randomly assigned to groups thereby naturally controlling for any confounds, ANCOVA should reveal more precise results (i.e., a smaller error term and thus a larger, more significant F-test). Keeping in mind that the data we are analyzing are nonperimental, and with unequal sample sizes across groups, the ANCOVA results may not be as promising as we would like. In fact, due to the lack of experimental rigor in the design (i.e., no random assignment to groups or manipulation of the IV), results from both the ANOVA and the ANCOVA should both be viewed cautiously.

ANCOVA and Follow-up Tukey Tests

As shown in Table 5.6, the macro-level results for the ANCOVA are initially promising with $F(4,521) = 3.02$, $p = 0.0176$ for the main effect of STAGEA on CONSB, 6 months later. The ES for STAGEA can be calculated by the ratio of $SS_{STAGEA}/SS_{Total} = 5.280/373.405 = 0.014$, representing a small, univariate (or an unacceptably small multivariate) proportion of shared variance between stage of

IV.

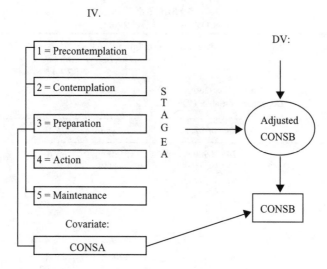

FIG. 5.1. ANCOVA with IV = STAGEA, covariate = CONSA, and DV = CONSB

condom use and perceived cons of condom use 6 months later. The proportion of shared variance between cons at $t1$ and cons at $t2$ is equal to $R^2 = \eta^2 = SS_{CONSA}/SS_{Total} = 113.19/373.405 = 0.30$, which indicates a very large univariate or multivariate ES for the covariate. Another way of assessing the ES for the covariate is to subtract the R^2 values between this ANCOVA that includes STAGEA and the covariate, CONSA, and the R^2 value from the ANOVA that included only the IV, STAGEA. This also reveals that $\eta^2_{STAGEA+CONSA} - \eta^2_{STAGEA} = 0.39 - 0.09 = 0.30$ is the unique ES for CONSA.

Figure 5.1 depicts the covariate, CONSA, predicting the DV, CONSB, with the IV, STAGEA, as the predictor to the adjusted CONSB that has removed the effects of the covariate.

It is now instructive to view the micro-results (i.e., means and Tukey tests) for the ANCOVA in Table 5.7. In Table 5.7, we see that the means and confidence intervals on CONSA across the 5 stages of condom use reveal relatively low values (i.e., close to 2 on a 5-point scale) with fairly small confidence intervals around the mean for individuals within stages 1 and 2 and moderately large confidence intervals for those in stages 3 to 5. This suggests that there is wider variation for those moving toward using condoms.

In contrast to the ANOVA micro-results, however, no significant differences are revealed with Tukey tests on CONSB, after controlling for levels of CONSA 6 months earlier. This can be seen in Table 5.7, where none of the p values for

TABLE 5.7
Micro-Level Follow-up Tukey Tests for ANCOVA

The GLM Procedure: Least Squares Means
Adjustment for Multiple Comparisons: Tukey-Kramer LSMEAN

STAGEA	CONSB LSMEAN	99% Confidence	Limits
1 = Precontemplation	2.171493	2.031365	2.311620
2 = Contemplation	2.056038	1.935708	2.176369
3 = Preparation	2.051618	1.847232	2.256004
4 = Action	1.873120	1.489926	2.256314
5 = Maintenance	1.862973	1.667728	2.058218

Least Squares Means for effect STAGEA Pr > |t| for H0:
LSMean(i)=LSMean(j) Dependent Variable: CONSB

i/j	1	2	3	4	5
1		0.4809	0.7232	0.3267	0.0101
2	0.4809		1.0000	0.7659	0.2007
3	0.7232	1.0000		0.8250	0.4139
4	0.3267	0.7659	0.8250		1.0000
5	0.0101	0.2007	0.4139	1.0000	

Least Squares Means for Effect STAGEA

i	j	Difference Between Means	Simultaneous 99% Confidence Limits for LSMean(i)-LSMean(j)	
1	2	0.115454	−0.116751	0.347659
1	3	0.119875	−0.194426	0.434175
1	4	0.298372	−0.219529	0.816273
1	5	0.308520	−0.000147	0.617187
2	3	0.004420	−0.296271	0.305112
2	4	0.182918	−0.326546	0.692382
2	5	0.193066	−0.100723	0.486854
3	4	0.178498	−0.370430	0.727425
3	5	0.188645	−0.167276	0.544566
4	5	0.010147	−0.529787	0.550082

the least squares means is less than our stringent alpha level of 0.01, although the difference between stages 1 and 5 comes close (i.e., $p = 0.0101$).

Because this is not an experimental design, it is difficult to come to definitive conclusions regarding the findings. It may be that the initial ANOVA findings of a (small to) medium ES (i.e., 0.09) was spurious and largely due to other confounds. Alternatively, it may be that there is truly a modest ES between STAGEA and CONSB, although the degree of correlation between the IV and covariate (i.e., $r = -0.30$: see correlation matrix presented earlier) was enough to cause some slight instability in the findings. These findings should be followed up in future work to understand better the nature of the links between the stages of condom use and the perceived disadvantages of condom use.

TABLE 5.8
Multiplicity, Background, Central, and Interpretation Themes Applied to ANCOVA

Themes	*ANCOVA*
Multiplicity Themes Note: + means multiplicity of theme pertains	+*Theory, hypotheses & empirical research* +*Controls*: With experimental design & covariate(s) +*Time Points*: Repeated measures +*Samples*: + Groups for IV(s) +*Measurements*: + IVs, 1 DV, & + Covariates
Background Themes	*Sample Data*: Random selection & assignment is best *Measures*: Grouping IVs, continuous covariate(s), continuous DV *Assumptions*: Normality, linearity, homoscedasticity, homogeneity of regressions *Methods*: Inferential with experimental design & assumptions
Central Themes	*Variance*: in DV *Covariance*: between DV & covariate(s) *Ratio*: Between groups/ within groups
Interpretation Themes **(Questions to Ask)**	*Macro*: F-test, ES $= \eta^2$ *Micro:* Tukey test of means, group comparisons Do groups differ after controlling for covariate? All variables reliable? Low-no correlation between IV & covariates? Correlation between DV & covariates? Are means significantly different, i.e., high between-group variance? Are groups sufficiently homogeneous, i.e., low within-group variance? Have possible confounds been considered?

SUMMARY

A summary of the multiplicity, background, central, and interpretation themes is presented in Table 5.8 as they apply to ANCOVA. Note that some of the information applies to the best use of ANCOVA (i.e., an experimental design with random assignment to groups). Thus, the nonexperimental application of ANCOVA that was just presented most likely would not exhibit some of the virtues that could be obtained in a more rigorous design.

REFERENCES

Cohen, J. (1988). *Statistical power analysis for the behavioral sciences.* San Diego, CA: Academic Press.

Cohen, J. (1992). A power primer. *Psychological Bulletin, 112*, 155–159.

Hair, J. F., Anderson, R. E., Tatham, R. L., & Black, W. C. (2004). *Multivariate data analysis* (6th ed.). Prentice Hall.

Pedhazur, E. J. (1997). *Multiple regression in behavioral research: Explanation and prediction* (3rd ed.). Belmont, CA: Wadsworth Publishing.

Prochaska, J. O., Velicer, W. F., Rossi, J. S., Goldstein, M. G., Marcus, B. H., Rakowski, W., Fiore, C., Harlow, L. L., Redding, C. A., Rosenbloom, D., & Rossi, S. R. (1994). Stages of change and decisional balance for 12 problem behaviors. *Health Psychology, 13*, 39–46.

Rutherford, A. (2001). *Introducing ANOVA and ANCOVA: A GLM approach.* Thousand Oaks, CA: Sage Publications.

SAS (1999). *The SAS system for windows.* Cary, NC: SAS Institute Inc.

Tabachnick, B.G., & Fidell, L.S. (2001). *Using multivariate statistics* (4th ed.). Boston: Allyn and Bacon.

Tukey, J.W. (1953). *The problem of multiple comparisons.* Unpublished manuscript, Princeton University (mimeo).

III

Matrices

6

Matrices and Multivariate Methods

Themes Applied to Matrices

This chapter focuses on matrices and how they relate to multivariate methods. As such, it is not a chapter on a specific method, but rather foundational information to help in understanding the calculations involved in many multivariate methods [e.g., multivariate analysis of variance (MANOVA), discriminant function analysis (DFA), canonical correlation (CC)]. Although a great deal could be written about matrices as is evident in several excellent sources (Harville, 1997; Namboordiri, 1984; Schott, 1997; Tabachnick & Fidell, 2001; Tatsuoka, 1971), in this chapter we focus on very basic information and calculations. The initial framework of presenting material within the 10 questions outlined at the end of the chapter on background themes will be modified somewhat to accommodate the topic of matrices.

WHAT ARE MATRICES AND HOW ARE THEY SIMILAR TO AND DIFFERENT FROM OTHER TOOLS?

A matrix is a way of organizing and manipulating information in a grid system consisting of rows and columns. Row and column numbers label cells of a matrix (e.g., position 4-3 is located in the 4th row, 3rd column). Knowledge of matrix calculations helps us to understand the complexity of multivariate statistics. This is particularly true because most multivariate methods cannot be fully described or analyzed with single variables or equations. Matrices provide a mechanism for handling multiple variables and equations. Computer programs use matrices for space allocation as well as computation.

Matrices can be viewed as cartons for carrying the many numbers involved in multivariate analyses. Just as scalar equations (e.g., $Y = mx + b$) organize numerical information into organized symbolic units, matrices serve this role for multivariate methods. There are similarities between single numbers and matrices, some of which are touched on later in this chapter. For example, the concept of adding or subtracting numbers has a direct parallel with matrices. We can always add or subtract matrices, as long as they have the same size (i.e., the same number of rows and the same number of columns). And, just as with individual numbers, the order of the numbers or matrices does not matter for addition, although it does matter for subtraction. Thus, when adding two numbers or two matrices, it does not matter which one comes first, whereas when subtracting two numbers or matrices the order is important. Another similarity between single numbers and matrices is the concept of dividing a number or matrix by itself. When dividing a single number by itself, the number 1 results. When dividing a matrix by itself, a matrix with 1s along the diagonal and 0s everywhere else (labeled an identity matrix) is the result. We will see more about this when discussing matrix division.

There are also clear differences between calculations involving single numbers and those involving matrices. Matrix multiplication and division are two kinds of calculations that are more complex and seemingly very different than when performing these operations on single numbers. Calculations with matrices also allow for concepts not even considered when using scalars. For example, we can calculate values such as a determinant, a trace, and eigenvalues of a matrix, all of which provide some indication of the variance of a matrix. These matrix concepts are discussed in more detail shortly.

WHAT KINDS OF MATRICES ARE COMMONLY USED WITH MULTIVARIATE METHODS?

There are several different types of matrices, each with different properties that are often seen in statistics. For each one, I mention the size and the physical characteristics. This includes making note of the number of rows and columns in a specific matrix, the shape (e.g., rectangular or square), and whether the matrix is symmetric (i.e., having the same elements in the upper right triangular portion as in the lower left triangular portion of a square matrix).

a. **Scalar**. This is the smallest matrix. It has one row and one column and is a single (1×1) number. Several examples of important scalars used in statistics include the mean, the number of variables (p), the sample size (N), and the sample size minus one ($N - 1$).

b. **Data matrix**. $\mathbf{X}$ is a ($N \times$ p) rectangular and nonsymmetrical matrix. A data matrix is used to store the information collected from N participants in the rows and on p variables stored in the columns. Thus, a data matrix with information from 100 participants and 20 variables would be a rectangular, nonsymmetric matrix with 100 rows and 20 columns.

c. **Vector**. A vector is usually a column (p × 1) or row (1 × p) from a larger matrix. For example, one column of a data matrix would provide values on one variable from all the N participants. On the other hand, one row of a data matrix would yield information on all the variables from one participant. A mean (M) vector can be created that contains the means of the p variables across all N participants (or across participants within a group). Mean vectors can then be used to create deviation scores if subtracted from original X scores (i.e., $X - M$).

d. **Sum of squares and cross-products matrix**. **SSCP** is a (p × p) square, symmetrical matrix and contains the numerators of the variance-covariance, Σ, matrix. Sums of squares (SS) are listed along the diagonal of the **SSCP** matrix and give the squared distance each score is from its mean. In the off-diagonals of the **SSCP** matrix, the cross products of the distances for pairs of variables are provided. We could create a **SSCP** matrix from calculating the squared deviations and cross products of an **X** matrix. In matrix format,

$$\mathbf{D'} \times \mathbf{D} = \mathbf{SSCP}, \tag{6.1}$$

where **D** = a deviation score matrix, **X** − **M**, and **D′** is the transpose of this deviation score matrix. A transpose of a matrix is formed by converting each column of a matrix to a corresponding row of the transposed matrix. Thus, the first column would become the first row; the second column would become the second row, and so on in a transposed matrix. This also could be visualized by toppling over a matrix on its right side (with the first row becoming the first column with the numbers in reverse order) and then flipping this from front to back (thus shifting the numbers to their correct position). The resulting **SSCP** matrix would have the SS for each variable along the diagonal and the cross products for each pair of variables in the corresponding off-diagonal cell (e.g., the cross product between variable 4 and variable 3 would be in the 4th row and the 3rd column). Though the concept of a **SSCP** matrix may sound a bit foreign, recognize that SS show up in other areas that examine the numerator of a variance term [e.g., analysis of variance (ANOVA) source table, where SS are divided by degrees of freedom to yield between-groups or within-groups variance]. The reason we do not see the cross product (i.e., **CP**) portion as often as SS is probably due to less use of multivariate methods that examine several continuous variables that may covary together as they predict one or more outcome variables. Let's turn to another matrix that builds on **SS** and **CP** values in multivariate methods.

e. **Variance-covariance matrix**. Σ is a (p × p) square and symmetric matrix from the population that has the variances of the p variables along the diagonal and covariances in the off-diagonals. In a sample, the variance-covariance matrix is referred to as **S**. Σ and **S** are sometimes called unstandardized correlation matrices and show how much two variables vary together using the original metric of the variables. Thus, values can range from zero to infinity for the variances along the diagonal, and from minus infinity to plus infinity for the covariances in the off-diagonals. A variance-covariance matrix can also be viewed as one step up from a **SSCP** matrix. That is, a sample **S** matrix is formed by placing the sum of squares divided by $N - 1$ along the diagonal for each variable, and placing the cross-products, (i.e., the sum of X minus the mean of X times Y minus the mean of Y), divided by $N - 1$ in the off-diagonals. Thus, the sample variance-covariance matrix equals:

$$\mathbf{S} = (1)/(N - 1) \times \mathbf{SSCP} \qquad (6.2)$$

The **SSCP** and **S** matrices are used in calculations for MANOVA and DFA (see Chapters 7 and 8), just as the SS and variances (between and within groups) are important for calculating ANOVA.

  f. **Correlation matrix.** **R** is a (p $\times$ p) square and symmetrical matrix. Ones are placed along the diagonal, with the off-diagonals showing the magnitude and direction of relationship between pairs of variables, using a standardized metric ranging from -1 to 1. Values close to the absolute value of 1 indicate strong relationships (i.e., variables vary together, rising and falling in similar patterns), and values close to zero indicate little to no relationship. A correlation, r, is calculated by: the covariance of X and Y, divided by the square root of the product of the variances of X and Y:

$$r = [(X - M_x)(Y - M_y)]/\sqrt{[(X - M_x)^2(Y - M_y)^2]} \qquad (6.3)$$

When there are more than 2 variables, it is helpful to store correlations (as in equation 6.3) in an **R** matrix, where each cell represents the correlation between the corresponding variables [e.g., $r(2, 1)$ is the correlation between variable 1 and variable 2]. There is a distinction between a correlation and covariance matrix. The correlation matrix tells us about the interpretable nature of the relationship between two variables whereas the covariance matrix tells us about how two variables vary using their original metric (e.g., inches, IQ points, etc.). Covariances are not easily interpretable as to the size or magnitude of the relationship. A correlation matrix is often used in multiple regression (see Chapter 4), CC (see Chapter 10), factor analysis and principal components analysis (see Chapter 11).

  g. **Diagonal matrix.** A diagonal matrix is a square, symmetric matrix with values on the diagonal and zeros on the off-diagonals. A common diagonal matrix is an identity matrix, **I**, which is the matrix parallel of the scalar, 1.0. As we will see later, **I** is also useful in verifying that we have found the inverse (i.e., divisor) of a matrix used in matrix division (i.e., $\mathbf{A}^{-1}\mathbf{A} = \mathbf{A}\,\mathbf{A}^{-1} = \mathbf{I}$, where $\mathbf{A}^{-1}$ is the inverse of the matrix **A**). Thus, if we divide a matrix by itself (i.e., multiply a matrix by its inverse), we will get an identity matrix, much like dividing a scalar by itself yields the number, 1.

WHAT ARE THE MAIN MULTIPLICITY THEMES FOR MATRICES?

Multiplicity themes do no directly apply to matrices since a matrix is just something that is involved when performing calculations with multivariate methods. The main point to remember regarding multiplicity and matrices is that matrices are capable of handling multiple pieces of information in easily summarized and manipulated form.

WHAT ARE THE MAIN BACKGROUND THEMES APPLIED TO MATRICES?

Similar to multiplicity themes, the notion of background themes does not directly apply to matrices, except to note that data considerations that pertain to individual variables can also apply to a set of variables within a matrix. We will get an introduction of how to analyze variables within a matrix in the next section.

WHAT KINDS OF CALCULATIONS CAN BE CONDUCTED WITH MATRICES?

Matrices can be manipulated by simple mathematical operations like addition, subtraction, multiplication and division:

a. **Adding and multiplying a matrix by a constant** is very simple, and the order is not important. Add (or multiply) the constant to (or by) each matrix element to form a new matrix with the same size but with different elements. Any mathematical operation done with a constant involves each value in the matrix. Using a small (2 × 2) matrix and a constant, 10, we can calculate the following:

Example of Multiplying a Matrix by a Constant

$$\begin{bmatrix} 2 & 4 \\ 3 & 5 \end{bmatrix} (10) = \begin{bmatrix} 2(10) & 4(10) \\ 3(10) & 5(10) \end{bmatrix} = \begin{bmatrix} 20 & 40 \\ 30 & 50 \end{bmatrix}$$

b. **Subtracting or dividing a matrix by a constant** is also straightforward, though the order is important. Subtract (or divide) a constant from (or into) each element in a matrix. The resulting matrix has the same size but changed elements:

Example of Dividing a Matrix by a Constant

$$\begin{bmatrix} 2 & 4 \\ 3 & 5 \end{bmatrix} \div (10) = \begin{bmatrix} 2/10 & 4/10 \\ 3/10 & 5/10 \end{bmatrix} = \begin{bmatrix} .2 & .4 \\ .3 & .5 \end{bmatrix}$$

c. **Adding matrices** requires that each matrix be the same size, that is, conformable. We can add two (2×2) matrices or two (4×3) matrices, but we cannot add a (2×2) matrix to a (4×3) matrix. Although the size is important, the order of operations is not important in adding matrices; that is, adding matrices $\mathbf{A} + \mathbf{B} = \mathbf{B} + \mathbf{A}$. To add matrices, simply add corresponding elements in the two matrices:

Example of Adding Two Matrices of the Same Size

$$\begin{bmatrix} 2 & 4 \\ 3 & 5 \end{bmatrix} + \begin{bmatrix} 5 & 1 \\ 7 & 6 \end{bmatrix} = \begin{bmatrix} 7 & 5 \\ 10 & 11 \end{bmatrix}$$

d. **Subtracting matrices** involves subtracting corresponding elements from two matrices of the same size. We can subtract two (2×2) matrices or two (4×3) matrices, but we cannot subtract a (2×2) matrix from a (4×3) matrix. Order *is* important when subtracting matrices. With matrices $\mathbf{A}$ and $\mathbf{B}$, $\mathbf{A} - \mathbf{B} \neq \mathbf{B} - \mathbf{A}$:

Example of Subtracting Two Matrices of the Same Size

$$\begin{bmatrix} 2 & 4 \\ 3 & 5 \end{bmatrix} - \begin{bmatrix} 5 & 1 \\ 7 & 6 \end{bmatrix} = \begin{bmatrix} -3 & 3 \\ -4 & -1 \end{bmatrix}$$

e. **Multiplying matrices** involves summing the products of corresponding elements in a row of the first matrix with those from a column of the second matrix. This requires that the number of columns in the 1st matrix equal the number of rows in the 2nd matrix. In other words, to multiply two matrices, the inside numbers must be the same. The size of the new matrix is given by the dimensions of the outside numbers, or the number of rows in the 1st matrix and the number of columns in the 2nd matrix. For example, a matrix of size (3×2) can be multiplied by a matrix of size (2×2) because the two inside numbers (i.e., 2 and 2) are the same. The dimensions of the resulting matrix will be (3×2) because these are the outside numbers (i.e., the number of rows in the 1st matrix by the number or columns in the 2nd matrix). When performing multiplication of matrices, use the row of the 1st matrix that corresponds with the desired row number of the element in the final product matrix. Also use the column of the 2nd matrix that corresponds with the column number for the relevant element of the final product matrix. Thus, when finding the (1, 2) element of a final product matrix, sum the products of each element in the 1st row of the first matrix times each element from the 2nd column of the second matrix.

Example of Multiplication of a (3 × 2) Matrix by a (2 × 2) Matrix, Yielding a (3 × 2) Matrix

$$\begin{bmatrix} 3 & 6 \\ 2 & 5 \\ 4 & 1 \end{bmatrix} \times \begin{bmatrix} 2 & 4 \\ 3 & 5 \end{bmatrix} = \begin{bmatrix} (3)(2)+(6)(3) & (3)(4)+(6)(5) \\ (2)(2)+(5)(3) & (2)(4)+(5)(5) \\ (4)(2)+(1)(3) & (4)(4)+(1)(5) \end{bmatrix} = \begin{bmatrix} 24 & 42 \\ 19 & 33 \\ 11 & 21 \end{bmatrix}$$

f. **Dividing matrices** is similar to dividing scalars (e.g., B/A) in logic, though the calculations are more complex with matrices. When dividing two matrices, we multiply the first matrix (e.g., **B**) by the inverse of the second matrix (e.g., **A**). If **A**, the matrix for which we need an inverse, is a (2 × 2) matrix, we can calculate the inverse by dividing the adjoint of matrix (see below) by the determinant (see below).

  i. **A determinant** is a single number that provides an index of the generalized variance of a matrix. It shows how much the variables of the matrix differ. For a correlation matrix, a determinant can range from 0 to 1.0. When variables are highly related, the determinant is close to zero, indicating that there is not much variation between the variables (i.e., the information is nearly redundant). For example, when examining two completely redundant variables (e.g., degrees in Fahrenheit and degrees in Centigrade) then the determinant would equal zero. When examining variables that are very different, the determinant is larger, reflecting the fact that the variables within the matrix are widely variant. For example, the determinant of a matrix with completely unrelated or orthogonal variables is 1.0 for a correlation matrix.

  The determinant of a 2 × 2 matrix equals the product of the main diagonal elements minus the product of the off-diagonals. When the 2 × 2 matrix is symmetric and the off-diagonals are less than or equal to the values along the diagonal, as with **SSCP**, **S**, and **R** matrices, the determinant should be a positive value indicating how much the variables differ in the kind of information they provide. If all the variables are completely orthogonal (i.e., unrelated), the determinant will be large. Conversely, if all the variables are perfectly collinear (i.e., redundant), the determinant will equal zero, indicating that there is no difference in the variance information provided by the separate variables. An unusual phenomenon occurs when a matrix is not positive definite (i.e., the matrix may not be symmetric and/or the off-diagonals may be larger than the diagonals). In the latter case, the determinant may be negative, which is difficult to interpret using the concept of a generalized variance because variance terms theoretically should be positive. Nonetheless, this is sometimes the case (see below), although hopefully not with the kinds of symmetric and positive definite (e.g., **SSCP**) matrices we often see in statistics.

Example of Calculating a Determinant

$$A = \begin{bmatrix} 2 & 4 \\ 3 & 5 \end{bmatrix}$$

Then, the determinant of $\mathbf{A} = |A| = (2 \times 5) - (4 \times 3) = 10 - 12 = -2$.

ii. We need to calculate the inverse of the divisor matrix whenever we need to divide matrices. The inverse is formed from dividing the **Adjoint** of a matrix by the determinant. To find an adjoint of a (2×2) matrix, switch the main diagonal elements, and keep off-diagonal elements in their original place, but multiply them by -1:

Example of Calculating an Adjoint

$$A = \begin{bmatrix} 2 & 4 \\ 3 & 5 \end{bmatrix} \text{ and the Adjoint of } \mathbf{A} = \begin{bmatrix} 5 & -4 \\ -3 & 2 \end{bmatrix}$$

g. To find **the inverse** of a matrix, multiply the adjoint of a matrix (switch the main diagonal elements, and multiply the off-diagonal elements by -1) by (1/determinant of the matrix):

Example of Calculating an Inverse (multiply adjoint matrix by one over determinant)

$$\begin{bmatrix} 5 & -4 \\ -3 & 2 \end{bmatrix} (1/-2) = \begin{bmatrix} 5/-2 & -4/-2 \\ -3/-2 & 2/-2 \end{bmatrix} = \begin{bmatrix} -2.5 & 2 \\ 1.5 & -1 \end{bmatrix} = \mathbf{A}^{-1}$$

To verify that we have calculated the correct Inverse of a matrix, we need to show that the original matrix multiplied by the inverse matrix, equals an **identity matrix (I**: a square matrix with 1s on the diagonal and zeroes elsewhere):

Example of Multiplying an Original Matrix by its Inverse, Yielding an Identity Matrix

$$\begin{bmatrix} 2 & 4 \\ 3 & 5 \end{bmatrix} \times \begin{bmatrix} -2.5 & 2 \\ 1.5 & -1 \end{bmatrix} = \begin{bmatrix} 2(-2.5) + 4(1.5) & 2(2) + 4(-1) \\ 3(-2.5) + 5(1.5) & 3(2) + 5(-1) \end{bmatrix}$$

$$= \begin{bmatrix} 1 & 0 \\ 0 & 1 \end{bmatrix} = \mathbf{I}$$

Having verified that we have the correct inverse for the divisor matrix, $\mathbf{A}$, we can now proceed to perform the division $\mathbf{B}/\mathbf{A} = (\mathbf{B})\,\mathbf{A}^{-1}$:

$$\begin{bmatrix} 5 & 1 \\ 7 & 6 \end{bmatrix} \times \begin{bmatrix} -2.5 & 2 \\ 1.5 & -1 \end{bmatrix} = \begin{bmatrix} 5(-2.5) + 1(1.5) & 5(2) + 1(-1) \\ 7(-2.5) + 6(1.5) & 7(2) + 6(-1) \end{bmatrix} = \begin{bmatrix} -11 & 9 \\ -8.5 & 8 \end{bmatrix}$$

HOW DO CENTRAL THEMES OF VARIANCE, COVARIANCE, AND LINEAR COMBINATIONS APPLY TO MATRICES?

The central themes of variance, covariance and linear combinations most certainly apply to matrices. First, the most central matrices used in multivariate methods involve some form of variances and covariances. For example, the **SSCP** matrix has the numerators of the variances (i.e., the sums of squares) along the diagonal and the numerators of the covariances (i.e., the cross products) along the off-diagonals. As shown previously, the variance-covariance matrix, $\mathbf{S}$, holds the variances along the diagonal and covariances in the off-diagonal. These matrices are directly analyzed in MANOVA and DFA (see Chapters 7 and 8, respectively) where we are interested in the ratio of between- over within-groups' variance-covariance matrices, just as we are interested in this ratio at a scalar level in ANOVA.

Linear combinations are also centrally linked to matrices in that we often need to combine multiple variables that are housed in matrices. These new (linear) combinations, which are simply composites of the original variables, often become the focal point in several multivariate methods [e.g., MANOVA, DFA, CC, and principal components analysis (PCA)]. As with many multivariate statistics, we are interested in analyzing the variance in a set of variables or linear combinations (see Chapter 2 regarding linear combinations).

The variances of linear combinations are called eigenvalues, which are actually just a redistribution of the original variances of the variables. There are usually p eigenvalues for each p × p matrix, where the sum of the eigenvalues is equal to the sum of the variances of the original matrix. Often we choose to examine only a portion of the original variance. This portion usually corresponds to the variances of the biggest linear combinations of the original variables. Thus, we would want to identify the largest eigenvalues, indicating that the corresponding linear combinations were retaining a good bit of the variance of the original variables. The linear combinations are formed to maximize the amount of information or variance that is taken from each of the individual variables to form a composite variable. **The specific amount of variance that is taken from each variable is called an eigenvector weight**. It is somewhat similar to an unstandardized multiple regression weight in telling us how much of a variable corresponds to the overall linear combination, allowing calculation of a determinant for any pxp matrix.

We can use an analogy with sandboxes to help describe the process with eigen-values and eigenvector weights. Imagine that the variance for each variable is contained in its own separate sandbox. We may want to form combinations of several variables to examine relationships between sets of variables. To do this, we can visualize a whole row of distinct sandboxes representing the variances for each of the variables with a whole row of empty and separate sandboxes behind them waiting to hold the variances of the new linear combinations that will be formed. Using information from eigenvector weights, we take a large (eigenvector weight) portion of sand from each of the first row of sandboxes and place it in the first back-row linear combination sandbox. The amount of sand in the first linear combination sandbox is indicated by its eigenvalue (i.e., the amount of variance in a linear combination). The process continues with more sand being drawn from the first row of sandboxes (i.e., the original variables' variance), which is placed in subsequent independent (i.e., orthogonal) back-row linear combination sandboxes. Remaining linear combination sandboxes contain less and less of the original sand because most of the information is placed in the first few linear combinations. Knowing that an eigenvalue is a variance for a linear combination, it is helpful to mention a single number that summarizes both eigenvalues and the variances in a matrix. This value is called a trace and is discussed next.

The sum of the variances or the sum of the eigenvalues is labeled a trace of a matrix. Thus, a trace tells us something about how much variance we have to ana-lyze in a matrix, just as with the set of eigenvalues of a matrix. We can write this as:

$$\text{trace}(\mathbf{A}) = \text{sum of diagonal elements of } \mathbf{A} = \mathbf{tr}(\mathbf{A}). \qquad (6.4)$$

If the matrix is a variance-covariance matrix, the trace provides a sum of all the variance in the set of variables. If the matrix is a correlation matrix, the trace is equal to the number of variables because each of the values along the diagonal is equal to 1.0. In both types of matrices, the trace gives us one way to summarize the amount of variance available in the set of variables, ignoring the (off-diagonal) covariance or correlation among the variables. Thus, the trace may not provide enough information about a set of variables if there is significant covariance among them, although it may be helpful when the variables are relatively orthogonal. Another index that may provide more information about the variance in a matrix than a trace does is discussed next.

Another useful operation is to calculate the determinant of a matrix by the product of the eigenvalues. Thus, if we knew all the p eigenvalues of a p × p matrix, we could multiply all of them and find the determinant. This would provide useful information about how much the set of variables provided relatively separate, nonredundant information (as with a large determinant), or whether we just had a set of highly redundant variables (yielding a small determinant that approached zero in value). Although it is beyond the scope of this chapter to go into the calculations for eigenvalues, they can easily be obtained from most factor analysis programs, allowing calculation of a determinant for any p × p matrix.

WHAT ARE THE MAIN THEMES NEEDED TO INTERPRET MATRIX RESULTS AT A MACRO-LEVEL?

When analyzing several variables, it is necessary to summarize results in terms of matrices instead of single numbers. At a macro-level, we would like to be able to examine some ratio of between over within information and assess whether it is significant. For example, in MANOVA (discussed in Chapter 7), we can look at the ratio of between-group over within-group SSCP matrices, just as with ANOVA we examine the ratio of between-group over within-group sums of squares. A problem with forming a ratio of matrices is that it yields another matrix that is not as easily summarized as a single number, such as the F-ratio in ANOVA. To address this, several suggestions have been offered to summarize matrices and ratios of matrices. In Chapter 7, we discuss indices that involve traces, eigenvalues, or determinants to summarize the variance in MANOVA.

For the time being, it is useful to realize that conceptually we are examining very similar ratios, whether using simple scalars (as with SS and MS in ANOVA) or larger matrices (as with the **SSCP** and **S** in MANOVA). When we ascertain that the ratio of between over within variance-covariance matrices indicates significant differences on some linear combinations of the variables, we can then proceed to examine where the specific differences lie.

WHAT ARE THE MAIN THEMES NEEDED TO INTERPRET MATRIX RESULTS AT A MICRO-LEVEL?

Much as with multiple regression (MR) and analysis of covariance (ANCOVA), we often examine either weights or means to assess the micro-aspects of an analysis. When analyzing weights in several multivariate methods (e.g., see DFA, CC, PCA in Chapters 8, 10, and 11, respectively), we are often analyzing some function of what are called eigenvectors of a matrix. Eigenvectors are simply vectors of weights that inform us how much of a variable is used in forming new linear combinations of the original variables. As with eigenvalues, we will not be working directly with calculations that form eigenvectors. When discussing DFA, CC, and PCA we will have occasion to see eigenvector weights, which are somewhat analogous to unstandardized regression weights in MR.

The main thing to take from this discussion is that one way to manage a large set of variables is to store them in a matrix. Then, to try and summarize the essence of a matrix, we can form linear combinations of the variables by scooping out eigenvector weight portions of the original variables and putting them into new composite variables. The variances of these new linear combination variables, as we have just mentioned, are called eigenvalues, which are simply redistributed variances from the original matrix of variables.

WHAT ARE SOME QUESTIONS TO
CLARIFY THE USE OF MATRICES?

a. **Under what circumstances would we subtract a constant from a matrix (especially in social sciences)?**

One example is when we have data and want to remove an error in measurement. Another example is when we want to subtract the mean from each score.

b. **What is the interrelationship of SSCP, covariance, and correlation matrices, i.e., how do we proceed from one matrix to the next.**

To begin calculating any of the (p × p) symmetric matrices that provide information on how variables vary and covary, begin with a data matrix. From a data matrix, calculate the mean of each (column) variable and insert the means into a row vector that is duplicated N times, so that there is the same row of means for each of the N participants. From the matrix of means, $\mathbf{M}$, create a deviation score matrix, $\mathbf{D}$, of $\mathbf{X}$ minus $\mathbf{M}$; then calculate a matrix of sums of squares and cross products by multiplying the transpose of the deviation score matrix, $\mathbf{D}'$, by the original deviation score matrix, $\mathbf{D}$ (i.e., $\mathbf{D}'\,\mathbf{D} = \mathbf{SSCP}$). Divide the elements in the **SSCP** matrix by $N - 1$ (sample size minus 1), which results in a sample variance-covariance matrix, $\mathbf{S}$. Divide the elements in $\mathbf{S}$ by the square root of the products of the individual variances of X and Y to get a correlation matrix, $\mathbf{R}$.

Given the above steps, it is still important to reiterate the relationship among these matrices. The $\mathbf{S}$ matrix is a square, symmetric matrix with variances on the diagonal, where a variance equals the sum of squares divided by $N - 1$, and covariances on the off-diagonals, where a covariance equals the cross-product of the deviation scores for two variables divided by $N - 1$. If we already have the $\mathbf{S}$ matrix and know $N - 1$, we can find the **SSCP** matrix by multiplying $\mathbf{S}$ by $N - 1$.

We can always calculate $\mathbf{R}$ from the $\mathbf{S}$ matrix, remembering that we are essentially standardizing the unstandardized $\mathbf{S}$ matrix by doing so. Take each element of $\mathbf{S}$, and divide it by the square root of the respective variances. This results in a matrix with ones on the diagonal (i.e., the variance, divided by the square root of the squared variance for a variable) and correlations on the off-diagonals (i.e., the covariance divided by the square root of the product of the variance of the first variable by the variance of the second variable).

c. **Why and when would we divide the between groups variance matrix by the within groups variance matrix?**

A ratio of between-group to within-group variance is central to ANOVA, ANCOVA, MANOVA, and MANCOVA. With the former two methods, this ratio involves a single number (i.e., the F-test). In the latter two procedures, the ratio forms a matrix that still needs to be summarized further (e.g., by using traces, determinants, or eigenvalues). Thus, this ratio is a common theme in group-difference statistics, allowing us to see if the means on one or more dependent variables across groups vary more than the individual scores within each group for the dependent variable. We would want this to be true, i.e., have greater variance between means than scores, in a study in which the groups are expected to reveal very different scores on the dependent variables.

   d. **How is the concept of orthogonality related to the concept of a determinant?**

   Orthogonality plays a role in the discussion of matrices. Total orthogonality in a correlational matrix would result in the largest possible attainable matrix determinant (i.e., 1.0). Total collinearity in a correlation matrix would result in the smallest possible correlational determinant (i.e., 0). The former would indicate that each of the variables provides very different information. In contrast, the later matrix has completely redundant information and thus a determinant of zero.

   Knowledge of the degree of relatedness among variables, as indicated by a determinant, often is used in behavioral science to understand the underlying structure of a data matrix. When a matrix has a determinant of zero, we cannot find an inverse for this matrix because anything divided by zero is undefined mathematically. Thus, it would not be useful to study variables that are completely redundant because they would result in a determinant of zero.

   e. **What is the relationship of generalized variance to orthogonality?**

   Generalized variance is a general estimate of how unique each measure is. Orthogonality occurs when measures are completely independent or unrelated. When measures are orthogonal, there will be huge generalized variance because the variables are completely unrelated.

WHAT IS AN EXAMPLE OF APPLYING MATRICES TO A RESEARCH QUESTION?

The topic of matrices and multivariate methods can become very tedious and abstract if it is not anchored in a clear application. To illuminate some of the ideas discussed here, we now turn to a very simplified example of examining the relationship between two variables, stage of readiness for condom use (STAGE) and the self-efficacy for condom use (CONSEFF). Though an actual study probably would include several other variables, and most likely a fairly large sample size, we limit our example to the two variables with data from only five participants. Though it is somewhat artificial, it is instructive for highlighting several of the concepts and calculations already discussed regarding matrices. As with previous examples, the theory that informs this example is drawn from the transtheoretical model of change, particularly as it applies to sexual risk taking and HIV prevention (e.g., Prochaska, Redding, et al., 1994; Prochaska, & Velicer, 1997; Prochaska, Velicer, et al., 1994).

   We could begin by featuring two important *scalars* in this example: $N = 5$, and $p = 2$. We could then provide a data matrix, $\mathbf{X}$, which would provide data from five participants in each of the five rows on two variables in each of the two columns:

Example of a (5 × 2) Data Matrix for Stage of Condom Use and Condom Self-Efficacy with $N = 5$

$$\begin{bmatrix} 4 & 2 \\ 3 & 2 \\ 1 & 2 \\ 5 & 3 \\ 2 & 1 \end{bmatrix}$$

We could then calculate the means for STAGE and CONSEFF and insert them into a row *mean vector* that we duplicate for each participant. Then, a matrix of means would be formed from concatenating the N identical rows of means for the p variables. The mean for STAGE is formed by finding the average of the first column of **X** [i.e., $(4 + 3 + 1 + 5 + 2)/5 = 15/5 = 3$]; the mean for CONSEFF is the average of the second column of **X**, and is equal to 2.

Example of an ($N \times$ p) Mean Matrix for STAGE and CONSEFF:

$$\begin{bmatrix} 3 & 2 \\ 3 & 2 \\ 3 & 2 \\ 3 & 2 \\ 3 & 2 \end{bmatrix}$$

We might now want to calculate a deviation score matrix, **D**, to form the **SSCP** matrix, (i.e., **D' D = SSCP**).

Example of Calculating a Deviation Score Matrix, D

$$\begin{bmatrix} 4 & 2 \\ 3 & 2 \\ 1 & 2 \\ 5 & 3 \\ 2 & 1 \end{bmatrix} - \begin{bmatrix} 3 & 2 \\ 3 & 2 \\ 3 & 2 \\ 3 & 2 \\ 3 & 2 \end{bmatrix} = \begin{bmatrix} 1 & 0 \\ 0 & 0 \\ -2 & 0 \\ 2 & 1 \\ -1 & -1 \end{bmatrix} = \mathbf{D} = \text{deviation score matrix}$$

Example of Calculating a SSCP matrix from D' D

$$\begin{bmatrix} 1 & 0 & -2 & 2 & -1 \\ 0 & 0 & 0 & 1 & -1 \end{bmatrix} \times \begin{bmatrix} 1 & 0 \\ 0 & 0 \\ -2 & 0 \\ 2 & 1 \\ -1 & -1 \end{bmatrix} = \begin{bmatrix} 10 & 3 \\ 3 & 2 \end{bmatrix} = \mathbf{SSCP}$$

Thus, the above matrix shows the sum of squares for STAGE is 10 and the sum of squares for CONSEFF is 2. The off-diagonals are identical and indicate the cross-product between STAGE and CONSEFF.

We can now form a variance-covariance matrix, **S**, by multiplying the **SSCP** matrix by $1/(N-1)$. Remember that it does not matter whether we multiply the constant, $1/(N-1)$, before or after the **SSCP** matrix because it will yield the same matrix. Notice, below, that the variances for STAGE and CONSEFF (i.e., 2.5 and 0.5, respectively) are along the diagonal, and the covariance between STAGE and CONSEFF (i.e., 0.75) is in the off-diagonal. Remember further that we cannot interpret the magnitude of the relationship between STAGE and CONSEFF by examining the covariance, although we can interpret the standardized covariance, or correlation, shortly when we calculate the correlation matrix, **R.**

Example of Calculating an S Matrix by Multiplying SSCP by $1/(N-1)$

$$\begin{bmatrix} 10 & 3 \\ 3 & 2 \end{bmatrix} \times 1/(5-1) = \begin{bmatrix} 10/4 & 3/4 \\ 3/4 & 2/4 \end{bmatrix} = \begin{bmatrix} 2.50 & 0.75 \\ 0.75 & 0.50 \end{bmatrix} = \mathbf{S}$$

We can now calculate the correlation matrix, **R**, by dividing the elements in the **S** matrix by the square root of the product of respective variances.

Example of Calculating an R Matrix from an S Matrix

$$\begin{bmatrix} 2.50/\sqrt{(2.5)(2.5)} & 0.75/\sqrt{(2.5)(0.5)} \\ 0.75/\sqrt{(2.5)(0.5)} & 0.50/\sqrt{(0.5)(0.5)} \end{bmatrix} = \begin{bmatrix} 1.00 & 0.75/1.118 \\ 0.75/1.118 & 1.00 \end{bmatrix}$$

$$= \begin{bmatrix} 1.00 & 0.67 \\ 0.67 & 1.00 \end{bmatrix} = \mathbf{R}$$

From the correlation matrix, we are free to interpret the magnitude and direction of the relationship between STAGE and CONSEFF as a moderately strong and positive correlation (i.e., $r = 0.67$).

Having calculated a number of important matrices with these data, it is instructive to perform several additional calculations to highlight some of the other matrix concepts. For example, we could calculate the determinant or generalized variance of the **R** matrix by the following:

determinant of R $= (1.0)(1.0) - (0.67)(0.67) = 1 - 0.4489 = \mathbf{0.5511}.$

This suggests that there is some moderately sized generalized variance between the variable STAGE and the variable CONSEFF. Remember that if the two variables were completely redundant, the determinant would be zero. If the two variables were completely orthogonal, the determinant would equal 1.0. Thus, the value 0.55 indicates that the two variables in the current **R** matrix are approximately midway between completely redundant and completely orthogonal.

It also would be a good exercise to calculate the inverse of our **R** matrix, remembering that this is formed from dividing the adjoint of **R** by the determinant of **R**.

Example of Calculating an Inverse for R

$$(1/0.5511) \times \text{adjoint of } \mathbf{R} = \begin{bmatrix} 1.00/0.5511 & -0.67/0.5511 \\ -0.67/0.5511 & 1.00/0.5511 \end{bmatrix}$$

$$= \begin{bmatrix} 1.81455 & -1.21575 \\ -1.21575 & 1.81455 \end{bmatrix} = \mathbf{R}^{-1}$$

We can verify that this is indeed the inverse of **R** by multiplying $\mathbf{R}^{-1}$ by **R** to yield an Identity matrix, **I**.

Example of Calculating R R^{-1} = I

$$\begin{bmatrix} 1.00 & 0.67 \\ 0.67 & 1.00 \end{bmatrix} \begin{bmatrix} 1.81455 & -1.21575 \\ -1.21575 & 1.81455 \end{bmatrix} = \begin{bmatrix} 1.00 & 0.00 \\ 0.00 & 1.00 \end{bmatrix} = \mathbf{I}$$

Finally, it would be helpful to also know the eigenvalues for the **R** matrix and verify that the sum of the eigenvalues is equal to the trace of **R**, and also show that the product of the eigenvalues is equal to the determinant of **R**. Using the PROC FACTOR routine in the SAS computer program, the two eigenvalues for the **R** matrix are 1.67 and 0.33. We can now show that the sum of the eigenvalues is equal to the trace of **R**.

Example of Calculating the Sum of the Eigenvalues = Trace of R

sum of the eigenvalues $= (1.67 + 0.33) = $ trace $\mathbf{R} = (1.0 + 1.0) = 2.0$

We can conclude by showing that the product of the eigenvalues equals the determinant of the matrix.

Example of Calculating the Product of the Eigenvalues = the Determinant of R

product of the eigenvalues $= (1.67)(0.33) = $ determinant of $\mathbf{R} = 0.5511$.

SUMMARY

In conclusion, we have outlined a number of matrices that are commonly used in multivariate methods, along with some basic calculations involving matrices. Examples of matrices include a simple (1×1) scalar matrix, such as N or p,

TABLE 6.1
Summary of Matrix Concepts

Concepts	Description
Scalar	(1×1) matrix or number (e.g., N, p, M)
Data matrix	$(N \times p)$ **X** matrix with N rows and p columns
Vector	$(p \times 1)$ column or $(1 \times p)$ row of a matrix
SSCP matrix	$(p \times p)$ square, symmetric matrix with sums of squares on the diagonal and cross-products on the off-diagonals
S matrix	$(p \times p)$ square, symmetric matrix with variances on the diagonal and covariances on the off-diagonals
R matrix	$(p \times p)$ square, symmetric matrix with 1s on the diagonal and correlations ranging from -1 to $+1$ on the off-diagonals
I matrix	Square, Symmetric matrix with 1s on the diagonal and 0s on the off-diagonals. It is the matrix parallel of the scalar "1"
Transpose	Matrix formed by exchanging rows (for **A**) for columns (in **A**$'$)
Eigenvalue	Variance of a linear combination; the sum of the eigenvalues = the trace of the original matrix
Eigenvector weights	Coefficients that indicate how much variance to extract from a variable when forming a linear combination
Adjoint	Matrix formed by exchanging the diagonal elements and multiplying off-diagonals by -1 in a (2×2) matrix
Determinant	Generalized variance of a matrix (ranging from 0 to 1 for **R**) equal to the product of the eigenvalues of a matrix
Inverse	A "divisor" matrix used in dividing a matrix. In a (2×2) matrix, this equals the adjoint divided by the determinant of a matrix
Trace	Sum of the diagonal elements of a matrix

TABLE 6.2
Summary of Matrix Calculations

Calculation	Description
Adding a constant	Adding a single number to each element of a matrix (e.g., adding 10 points to all students' exam score ☺)
Subtracting a constant	Subtracting a single number from each element of a matrix (e.g., subtracting the mean to form deviation scores)
Multiplying by a constant	Multiplying each element in a matrix by a single number (e.g., multiplying an **S** matrix by "$N-1$" to yield a **SSCP** matrix)
Dividing by a constant	Dividing each element of a matrix by a single number (e.g., dividing the **SSCP** matrix by "$N-1$" to yield an **S** matrix)
Adding matrices	Adding each element in one matrix to the corresponding element in another matrix of the same size (e.g., adding matrices of exam scores from 2 portions of a test to yield total scores)
Subtracting matrices	Subtracting each element in one matrix from the corresponding element in another matrix of the same size (e.g., subtracting a matrix of means from an **X** matrix to yield a deviation matrix, **D**)
Multiplying matrices	Summing the products of the elements of one row with the elements of a column (e.g., multiplying **D**$'$ by **D** to yield **SSCP**)
Dividing matrices	Multiplying a matrix by the inverse of the divisor matrix (e.g., dividing a matrix by its inverse to yield an **I** matrix)

an ($N \times$ p) data matrix, **X**, and a vector that is simply a row or column from a larger matrix. We also looked at the progression from the **SSCP**, **S**, and **R** matrices each depicting the relationship between variables in increasingly standardized and interpretable form.

We also showed how to calculate various matrix concepts such as the determinant, the adjoint, the inverse, the trace, and the identity matrix. Finally, we found that we can have a computer calculate the eigenvalues of a matrix, which are useful in calculating the determinant and verifying the trace of a matrix.

A summary of matrix concepts is provided in Table 6.1, with a summary of matrix calculations in Table 6.2. In subsequent chapters, we return to some of these concepts and calculations when discussing various multivariate methods that make use of them.

REFERENCES

Harville, D. A. (1997). *Matrix algebra from a statistician's perspective*. New York: Springer.

Namboordiri, K. (1984). *Matrix algebra: An introduction*. Beverly Hills, CA: Sage Publications.

Prochaska, J. O., Redding, C. A., Harlow, L. L., Rossi, J. S., & Velicer, W. F. (1994). The transtheoretical model and HIV prevention: A review. *Health Education Quarterly, 21*, 45–60.

Prochaska, J. O., & Velicer, W. F. (1997). The transtheoretical model of health behavior change (invited paper). *American Journal of Health Promotion, 12*, 38–48.

Prochaska, J. O., Velicer, W. F., Rossi, J. S., Goldstein, M. G., Marcus, B. H., Rakowski, W., Fiore, C., Harlow, L. L., Redding, C. A., Rosenbloom, D., & Rossi, S. R. (1994). Stages of change and decisional balance for 12 problem behaviors. *Health Psychology, 13*, 39–46.

Schott, J. R. (1997). *Matrix analysis for statistics*. New York: Wiley.

Tabachnick, B. G., & Fidell, L. S. (2001). *Using multivariate statistics* (4th ed.: Appendix A, pp. 908–917). Boston: Allyn and Bacon.

Tatsuoka, M. (1971). *Multivariate analysis: Techniques for educational and psychology research*. New York: Wiley.

IV

Multivariate Group
Methods

7

Multivariate Analysis of Variance

Themes Applied to Multivariate Analysis of Variance (MANOVA)

MANOVA is the first multivariate method we cover that allows for multiple dependent variables. The previous presentation on intermediate methods as well as the topic of matrices discussed in Chapter 6 help in forming a base from which to discuss the rigorous capabilities of MANOVA. As we shall see shortly, background, central, and multiplicity themes also apply to MANOVA, similar to yet extending from what we saw with the methods of multiple regression (MR) and analysis of covariance (ANCOVA).

WHAT IS MANOVA AND HOW IS IT SIMILAR TO AND DIFFERENT FROM OTHER METHODS?

MANOVA is a group difference method (e.g., Grimm & Yarnold, 1995; Maxwell & Delaney, 2003; Tabachnick & Fidell, 2001), extending analysis of variance (ANOVA) to allow for *several* continuous dependent variable (DVs). In MANOVA, we ask whether there are significant group differences on the best linear combinations of our continuous DVs. As with ANOVA and ANCOVA, MANOVA is a useful procedure whenever we have limited resources and want to identify which groups may need specific treatments or interventions. MANOVA can be used to identify which and how groups differ as well as on which DVs.

In ANOVA, we allow one or more categorical independent variables (IVs), each with two or more groups, and one continuous DV. With MANOVA, we allow the same structure of IVs and *two or more* DVs. Thus, MANOVA allows for a much more realistic appraisal of group differences than does ANOVA. MANOVA also can be extended to incorporate one or more covariates, essentially becoming an ANCOVA that allows for two or more (continuous) DVs [i.e., multivariate analysis of covariance (MANCOVA)]. MANOVA is somewhat similar to discriminant function analysis (DFA) and logistic regression (LR), which will be discussed in upcoming chapters (8 and 9, respectively), in that all three methods include at least one major categorical variable. In MANOVA, the major categorical variable is on the independent side, whereas with DFA and LR, the DV is categorical.

MANOVA differs from purely correlational methods such as MR and other correlational methods discussed later [i.e., canonical correlation (CC), principal components analysis (PCA), and factor analysis (FA)] in that with MANOVA we are very interested in assessing the *differing means between groups,* whereas with the other methods the focus is not on the means but on *correlations or weights between variables* (see Chapters 10 and 11, respectively).

WHEN IS MANOVA USED AND WHAT RESEARCH QUESTIONS CAN IT ADDRESS?

There are three main uses of MANOVA, which are presented below:

a. **MANOVA can be used in an experimental design** to assess group differences on a set of DVs that are usually conceptually related. For example, at the beginning of an experimental design assessing reading, we could examine whether there are any significant differences between treatment and control groups (i.e., IV = treatment condition with two levels) on several (dependent) background variables (e.g., age, education, income, pretest scores). In this case, we would hope that there were *not* any significant differences because we would like to have comparable groups before applying the treatment. At the end of the study, we would want to conduct another MANOVA, also using the same IV (i.e., treatment condition), and with two or more DVs (e.g., reading comprehension, vocabulary). In the latter MANOVA, if we found there were significant differences between groups on the best linear combination of the DVs, we could conclude that they were due to the treatment (given a large, random sample with random assignment to groups).

b. **MANOVA can be used to analyze repeated measures designs** where there may be several time points collected on one or more DVs (e.g., examine group differences on smoking levels at three different time points). In this example, time is the IV with levels representing the separate time points, and the set of DVs is the single DV that is measured k (i.e., the number of levels or groups in the IV) times. This is also called a within-groups design as the analysis is assessed within a single group, across time. It also could be referred to as a dependent MANOVA because the scores at each time point depend on the previous time point with the same (within-group) sample providing repeated measures across time.

c. **MANOVA can be used in a nonexperimental design** to assess differences between two or more intact groups, on two or more DVs (e.g., examine differences between men and women on several substance use variables). In this example, the IV would be gender with several DVs (e.g., alcohol use, marijuana use, hard drug use). Even if we found significant differences between gender groups, it would be impossible to attribute causality, especially because we did not manipulate the IV and most likely did not build in adequate control for confounding variables. Nonetheless, this form of MANOVA is often used with results interpreted more descriptively than inferentially.

WHAT ARE THE MAIN MULTIPLICITY THEMES FOR MANOVA?

There are a number of ways multiplicity themes apply to MANOVA. As with all the methods we address here, it is important to consider multiple theories and empirical studies before embarking on a study using MANOVA. These would inform our study of group differences, hopefully suggesting several relevant DVs with which to test meaningful hypotheses. When at all possible, it would be preferable to experimentally manipulate the categorical IV and randomly assign participants to a few, well-selected groups with a few relevant DVs. If too many groups or variables are included, it becomes difficult to find significance for any of them. This could be due to the reduced degrees of freedom in the error term as well as the possibility of less actual difference between too many groups or variables. For example, if a sports psychologist wanted to examine the effect of levels of exercise on relevant outcome variables it probably would be best to limit to only a few distinct levels of the IV (e.g., no exercise, 2 hours, or 5 or more hours per week) and a few outcomes (e.g., well-being, weight, stress levels). If more groups were added (e.g., 1 hour, 3 hours, 4 hours) to these other three groups, it would become very difficult to find group differences because there would not be very much separation between groups. Likewise, if more DVs were added (e.g., self-esteem, body mass, relaxation), the set of variables most likely would become redundant, causing instability in the findings and less significance than with fewer, more distinct variables.

A good guideline is to strive for little overlap among groups or continuous variables within a side (e.g., independent or dependent) and strive for moderate overlap across sides (from independent to dependent). This would prevent collinearity and maximize effect sizes.

Another multiplicity theme is to consider adding covariates, thus creating a MANCOVA that statistically controls for possible confounds. This is especially preferable in designs that do not build in experimental control. If groups can be statistically equated on several relevant variables, there is better opportunity to isolate an effect, separate from other background variables (i.e., covariates).

Although this is not always possible, it is a good idea to consider collecting data over multiple time points, perhaps assessing an independent grouping variable initially, along with several potential covariates and pretest scores and then assess dependent outcomes at a follow-up time period. If clear effect sizes emerge across time, there is greater evidence as to the temporal ordering of the variables.

Another way to build multiplicity is to test hypotheses on more than one sample. If comparable findings occur across different samples, this would extend the generalizability of the study. Even if findings are not completely replicated across samples, information can be gleaned on which sample characteristics might lead to specific findings. This could be done by randomly splitting a large sample in half and comparing group differences across samples.

Finally, there may well be a curvilinear relationship between multiplicity and scientific rigor. Adding more than one theory, study, IV, DV, or method, for example, is advisable to fully tap the phenomenon under study, although including too many may muddy the findings.

WHAT ARE THE MAIN BACKGROUND THEMES APPLIED TO MANOVA?

As with all statistical methods, it is useful to consider several background themes for MANOVA. First, we would want to ensure that we have a fairly large $(N \times p)$ data matrix that includes at least one categorical grouping IV, several continuous outcome variables, and possibly several continuous covariates. When covariates are added, this procedure is labeled as MANCOVA. Similar to ANCOVA, we would want to be sure that any covariate was reliable and essential to the study (i.e., significantly correlated with one or more of the dependent variables). To make findings more robust, we would want to attempt to have approximately equal numbers of participants for each group. It also would be useful to consider a power analysis (e.g., Cohen, 1988) to make sure enough participants were included for each group to find the desired effect size.

Kraemer and Thiemann (1987) provide an overview of power calculations for several simple designs. Using their guidelines, we could extrapolate how to conduct power calculations for a simple MANOVA design based on suggestions for a two-group independent design. This would involve the following steps:

a. **Estimate the desired standardized difference between groups.** This is sometimes referred to as either Cohen's d or Glass's effect size. In either case, it is calculated as follows:

$$D = M_1 - M_2/\text{pooled } s \qquad (7.1)$$

where M_i is the mean of a DV in group i, and S is the average or pooled standard deviation across groups.

b. **Calculate the critical effect size:**

$$\Delta = d/(d^2 + 1/qr)^{1/2} \tag{7.2}$$

where d = Cohen's d as in equation 1, q = proportion of participants in group 1, and r = proportion of participants in group 2.

c. **Estimate the sample size needed per DV:**

$$N = \nu + 2 \tag{7.3}$$

where ν is an estimate of sample size found in power tables (e.g., Cohen, 1988; Kraemer & Thiemann, 1987), given a specific power (e.g., 80%), alpha level (e.g., 0.05), and critical effect size.

As an example, if we expected a medium Cohen's d effect size of 0.5, with an equal proportion of participants per group (i.e., $q = r = 0.5$), 80% power, alpha $= 0.05$, and a two-tailed test, we would calculate:

$$\Delta = 0.5/(0.25 + 1/.25)^{1/2} = 0.5/(4.25)^{1/2} = 0.5/2.06 = 0.24.$$

Looking in the master table of Kraemer and Thiemann (1987), we find that $\nu = 133$. Thus, we would need an approximate sample size of:

$$N = 133 + 2 = 135.$$

With two groups, we should try to have at least 68 participants per group to detect a medium effect size with 80% power (i.e., that would correctly reject the null hypothesis of no effects 80% of the time), and with only a 5% chance of making a Type I error. With more than one outcome variable used in MANOVA, it would be advisable to include even more than the minimum suggested sample size per group.

After estimating sample size and collecting data to test hypotheses of group differences on two or more DVs, it also would be helpful to calculate basic descriptive statistics to show the means and standard deviations for the variables involved. It also would be helpful to calculate reliability coefficients for all variables and to check whether assumptions were met. These are the same as those for MR and include normality, linearity, and homoscedasticity. These assumptions could be at least preliminarily, assessed with an examination of skewness, kurtosis, and bivariate scatter plots. If covariates are included (i.e., a MANCOVA is conducted), then, similar to ANCOVA, the assumption of homogeneity of regressions must be met; that is, there should be no interaction between a covariate and a grouping variable.

WHAT IS THE STATISTICAL MODEL THAT IS TESTED WITH MANOVA?

The theoretical model of MANOVA is similar to the ANOVA theoretical model where:

$$Yi = \mu_{yi} + \tau + E \tag{7.4}$$

where Yi is a continuous DV, μ_{yi} is the grand mean of the ith DV, τ is the treatment effect, and E is error variance.

For MANOVA, we also have to include the following to recognize that we are forming linear combinations of the dependent variables:

$$V_i = b1Y1 + b2Y2 + \cdots + bpYp \tag{7.5}$$

where V_i is the ith linear combination, bi is the ith eigenvector weight, and Yi is the ith DV.

For a MANOVA, we can form one or more linear combinations, where the number is determined by:

$$\text{number of } V_i\text{s} = \text{minimum } (p, k - 1), \tag{7.6}$$

where p is the number of DVs, and k is the number of groups or levels of the IV. With only two groups, we will form only one (i.e., $2 - 1 = 1$) linear combination no matter how many DVs we have in our design.

In MANOVA, even though we are forming one or more linear combinations, each with a specific set of eigenvector weights (i.e., the b values in equation 7.5), we do not tend to focus on these combinations scores or weights until we get to DFA in the next chapter. For now, we also need to know how we are modeling group differences in MANOVA. Similar to ANOVA, we form a ratio of between-group variance over within-group variance except that, with MANOVA, we are now forming a ratio of variance-covariance (i.e., **S**) matrices. The between-group variance-covariance matrix could be labeled B, but to distinguish it from the un-standardized B regression weight in MR, this matrix is often labeled as **H** for the "hypothesis" matrix; the within-group variance-covariance matrix is often labeled **E** to represent error variance (Harris, 2001).

A ratio of variance matrices is then formed that is analogous to that found with the ratio of variance scalars in ANOVA:

$$\text{Between groups } \mathbf{S} \text{ matrix over error } \mathbf{S} \text{ matrix} = \mathbf{H}/\mathbf{E} = \mathbf{E}^{-1}\mathbf{H} \tag{7.7}$$

Remembering our matrix operations from Chapter 6, equation 7.7 is forming the familiar ratio of between or within groups variance. With MANOVA, however, the ratio involves matrices, and we need to form an inverse of the divisor ($\mathbf{E}$) matrix and then multiply this inverse by the dividend ($\mathbf{H}$) matrix. As we see later in the chapter, one of the challenges in conducting a MANOVA is summarizing the essence of this ratio of matrices with a single number that can be assessed for significance with an F-test. Several methods are suggested to summarize this matrix, including determinants, traces, and eigenvalues, all of which focus on variance information (see Chapter 6).

HOW DO CENTRAL THEMES OF VARIANCE, COVARIANCE, AND LINEAR COMBINATIONS APPLY TO MANOVA?

As with ANOVA, in MANOVA we focus on the ratio of the variance between means over the variance within scores. If this ratio is large, we can reject the null hypothesis of no significant differences between means. In addition to the variance of a single DV, as with ANOVA, in MANOVA we need to focus on p variances, one for each DV, as well as p (p − 1)/2 covariances among the p DVs. We store the variances and covariances in matrices.

Linear combinations are actually found for the matrix formed from the ratio of $\mathbf{E}^{-1}$ $\mathbf{H}$. With MANOVA, we are also interested in the eigenvalues of these linear combinations because they are used in forming some of the summary values of the $\mathbf{E}^{-1}$ $\mathbf{H}$ matrix before calculating an F-test. Remember that we can find as many linear combinations and eigenvalues as the minimum number of DVs or number of groups minus one. We see this more clearly in our example at the end of the chapter.

For now, it is important to realize that the concepts of variance and covariance are essential to an understanding of MANOVA, with the concept of linear combinations being relevant, although less central.

WHAT ARE THE MAIN THEMES NEEDED TO INTERPRET MANOVA RESULTS AT A MACRO-LEVEL?

As with ANOVA and ANCOVA, MANOVA results should be interpreted first at the macro-level. Similar to ANOVA and ANCOVA, we are first interested in whether there is a significant macro-level effect and the size of the effect, and second whether there are significant micro-level differences between pairs of groups. In addition, MANOVA is concerned about which DVs are showing significant differences across groups, adding a third, mid-level layer to the interpretation of results.

Several macro-assessment summary indices have been offered to summarize results for MANOVA. Probably the most widely used macro-assessment summary index is Wilks's (1932) lambda, which uses determinants to summarize the variance in the ratio of matrices formed in MANOVA. Wilks suggested that the determinant of the within-groups variance-covariance matrix over the determinant of the total (i.e., within plus between) variance-covariance matrix indicates how much of the variation and covariation between the grouping variable(s) and the continuous variables was unexplained. Thus, one minus the ratio of Wilks's lambda is a measure of the shared or explained variance between grouping and continuous variables. Two other macro-assessment summary indices incorporate the trace of a variance-covariance matrix to summarize group difference matrices. Hotelling's trace is simply the sum of the diagonal elements of the matrix formed from the ratio of the between-groups over the within-groups-variance-covariance matrix (i.e., $\mathbf{E}^{-1}\,\mathbf{H}$). Pillai's trace is the sum of the diagonal elements of the between-groups variance-covariance matrix over the total (i.e., between plus within) variance-covariance matrix (i.e., $[\mathbf{H}+\mathbf{E}]^{-1}\,\mathbf{H}$). A fourth macro-assessment summary is Roy's greatest characteristic root (GCR) (Harris, 2001). The GCR is actually the largest eigenvalue from the $\mathbf{E}^{-1}\,\mathbf{H}$ matrix, providing a single number that gives the variance of the largest linear combination from this matrix.

Below, I delineate further how to summarize macro-level information from MANOVA (and MANCOVA).

Significance Test

Each of the four main macro summary indices just described has an associated F-test for assessing whether group differences are significantly different from chance:

i. The most common macro summary index is *Wilks's (1932) lambda*, and its associated F-test. Wilks's lambda shows the amount of variance in the linear combination of DVs that is not explained by the IVs. Therefore, it is preferable to get low values for Wilk's lambda (closer to zero than 1). If the associated F-statistic is significant, we can conclude that there are significant differences between at least two groups on the linear combination of DVs. Wilks's lambda can be calculated as follows:

$$\Lambda = |\,\mathbf{E}\,|/|\,\mathbf{H}+\mathbf{E}\,| \qquad (7.8)$$

where | | stands for the determinant of the matrix inside the parallel lines.

ii. The second macro summary index is the *Hotelling-Lawley trace* and the associated F-test. This is formed by summing up the diagonal elements in the $\mathbf{E}^{-1}\,\mathbf{H}$ matrix (see equation 7.7):

$$\text{Hotelling-Lawley trace} = \text{tr}[\mathbf{E}^{-1}\,\mathbf{H}]$$

$$= \text{sum of eigenvalues of } \mathbf{E}^{-1}\,\mathbf{H} \qquad (7.9)$$

iii. A third macro-summary index is *Pillai's trace* and it's associated *F*-test. Pillai's trace is the sum of the diagonal values of the matrix formed from the ratio of the **H** over the **E** + **H** matrices:

$$\text{Pillai's trace} = \text{tr } [\mathbf{H}/(\mathbf{H} + \mathbf{E})]$$

$$= \text{sum of eigenvalues for } \mathbf{H}/(\mathbf{H} + \mathbf{E}) \qquad (7.10)$$

Pillai's trace has the advantage of being the most robust of the four summary indices when there are less-than-ideal conditions, such as unequal sample size or heterogeneity of variances. Pillai's trace also can be interpreted as the proportion of variance in the linear combination of DVs that is explained by the IV(s). Thus, it is intuitively meaningful.

iv. A fourth macro-summary index is called Roy's largest root or the GCR. Thus, this can be simply represented as follows:

$$\text{GCR} = \text{the largest eigenvalue of } \mathbf{E}^{-1} \mathbf{H} \qquad (7.11)$$

Effect Size

A common multivariate effect size for MANOVA is eta-squared:

$$(\eta^2) = (1 - \Lambda), \qquad (7.12)$$

where η^2 represents the proportion of variance in the best linear combination of DVs that is explained by the grouping IVs, and Λ represents Wilks's lambda. Eta-squared (η^2) can be interpreted with the multivariate guidelines of Cohen (e.g., 1992). Thus, a small effect size would be equal to about 0.02, a medium effect size would equal 0.13 or better, and a large effect size would be greater than or equal to about 0.26 (Cohen, 1992).

WHAT ARE THE MAIN THEMES NEEDED
TO INTERPRET MANOVA RESULTS
AT A MICRO- (AND MID-) LEVEL?

If the macro-level *F*-test is significant in MANOVA and there is a reasonable effect size, there are at least two more layers to interpret. Just as with ANOVA, this most likely involves micro-level significance tests of specific group differences and effect sizes for group means. But first, it is important to conduct a mid-level evaluation of the dependent variables.

a. **Follow-up analyses on the dependent variables** are conducted after finding a significant macro-level *F*-test. This can take several forms:

    i. Probably the most common follow-up to a significant MANOVA is to conduct a separate ANOVA for each DV. Researchers would hope to find a significant F-test for each DV, indicating that these variables each show significant differences across two or more groups.

    ii. As introduced in Chapter 5, another follow-up, sometimes conducted in lieu of a set of ANOVAs, is to perform a separate ANCOVA for each DV, using the remaining DVs as covariates in each analysis. This has been suggested by Bock (1966; Bock & Haggard, 1968) and is considered a step-down procedure. If these analyses revealed significant F-tests, it would suggest that there were significant group differences on a DV after partialing out any overlapping variance among the remaining continuous DVs used in the MANOVA. Thus, we could examine group differences for the unique portion of each DV that is purged of any relationship with other DVs. This provides a fairly rigorous assessment of group differences and is not often seen in the literature, possibly because of its difficulty in finding significant differences on such small, unique portions of the DVs.

    iii. Still another possible follow-up procedure after a significant macro-level F-test with MANOVA, is to conduct a single DFA with the same variables that were used in the MANOVA except that the roles (independent or dependent) are reversed. Thus, a DFA would use each of the continuous (dependent) variables from a MANOVA as the continuous IVs. The categorical (independent) grouping variable from MANOVA would now become the categorical DV in DFA. The goal would be to assess how each of the continuous variables discriminated among the groups of the DFA outcome variable. The standardized weights would be the focus in DFA, so that the continuous variable with the largest standardized weight would also be the variable that has the largest group differences on the categorical variable. In this way, we could assess which of the continuous variables are showing the clearest differences across groups without having to conduct separate (ANOVA or ANCOVA) analyses for each DV. Thus, the overall error rate is most likely smaller with a single DFA follow-up than with p follow-up ANOVAs or ANCOVAs, especially if the error rate was not adjusted (as with a Bonferroni approach).

    b. **Follow-up planned comparisons** (e.g., post hoc, simple effects, etc.) would be important micro-level assessment if there were more than two groups. These would provide a specific examination of which groups are showing differences on each of the DVs. Tukey (1953) honestly significant difference (HSD) tests between pairs of means would provide some protection for overall Type I error (i.e., rejecting Ho when it is true). Alternatively, a Bonferroni approach could be adopted whereby the total alpha was split among the number of pair-wise group tests. Still another possibility is to increase statistical power and reduce the probability of a Type II error (i.e., retaining Ho when it is false) by using an alpha level of 0.05. Researchers need to choose which error to protect, Type I or Type II.

   c. As with significance tests, **two levels (mid- and micro-level) of effect sizes can be examined after finding a significant macro-level effect in MANOVA:**

     i. A shared variance midlevel effect size (e.g., r^2 = sum of squares between groups divided by sum of squares within groups) could be calculated for each DV to assess the proportion of variance in common between that specific continuous variable and the grouping variable(s). Cohen's (1992) guidelines for univariate effects would apply here: 0.01 for a small effect, 0.06 for a medium effect, and about 0.13 or more for a large effect.

    ii. For MANOVA, Cohen's d can provide a micro-level effect size for the difference between a pair of means (e.g., Cohen, 1988, 1992), just as with ANOVA and ANCOVA. This is easily calculated with the formula in equation 7.1. The same values suggested for ANCOVA also apply for follow-up ANOVAs on each DV. Thus, a standardized difference of 0.20 is a small effect, a d of 0.50 is a medium effect, and 0.80 represents a large effect.

   d. Just as with univariate ANOVAs, or with intermediate ANCOVAs, **we can graph the means in MANOVA for each group** to provide a qualitative examination of specific differences between groups. Many computer programs allow this to be easily accomplished.

WHAT ARE SOME OTHER CONSIDERATIONS OR NEXT STEPS AFTER APPLYING THESE METHODS?

As with most analyses, it is important to ask whether a MANOVA design could allow for causal inferences. This would depend on the extent to which experimental design procedures were followed. Was the IV manipulated? Were participants from a large and representative sample randomly assigned to groups? Were possible confounds controlled for, either with an experimental design or with the inclusion of relevant covariates? If the answer is yes to each of these questions, a researcher is in a much better position to ascribe causality to the IV and to generalize beyond the specific sample. As with all research, results would be strengthened if the study were replicated in an independent sample. Variables also should be evaluated as to their reliability and validity as well as their relatively unique and nonredundant nature when compared with the full set of DVs.

WHAT IS AN EXAMPLE OF APPLYING MANOVA TO A RESEARCH QUESTION?

Here I present an example of MANOVA where the initial STAGEA of condom use is the IV (with five levels: precontemplation, contemplation, preparation, action, and maintenance of condom use), and there are several DVs: pros of condom use

TABLE 7.1
MANOVA Example Descriptive Frequencies

STAGEA	Frequency	Percent	Cumulative Frequency	Cumulative Percent
1 = Precontemplation	151	28.65	151	28.65
2 = Contemplation	204	38.71	355	67.36
3 = Preparation	70	13.28	425	80.65
4 = Action	20	3.80	445	84.44
5 = Maintenance	82	15.56	527	100.00

(PROSB), cons of condom use (CONSB), self-efficacy for condom use (CON-SEFFB), and psychosexual functioning (PSYSXB) assessed 6 months later. As with the MR and ANCOVA examples, this application draws on the theories of the transtheoretical model (e.g., Prochaska et al., 1994) and the multifaceted model of HIV risk (Harlow et al., 1993).

A caution before beginning analyses is that this application of MANOVA is not ideal as the levels of the IV are not manipulated but are intact stages in which people fall depending on the length of time for which they have used or considered using condoms. Still, it is worthwhile to examine the steps needed for a MANOVA as well as provide a brief interpretation of the output.

Output is provided below for several sets of analyses: A, descriptive statistics; B, correlations; C, MANOVA; D, ANOVAs; E, Tukey tests of HSDs between groups.

Descriptive Statistics

Table 7.1 presents the frequencies of participants at each of the five levels of the IV, STAGEA. Note that there is an imbalance in the number of participants per group. Most participants are in STAGEA 2 (contemplating condom use) or STAGEA 1 (precontemplation: not even considering condom use). Such unequal samples sizes across groups can reduce the power of a MANOVA (e.g., Kraemer & Thiemann, 1987). Still, we proceed with caution, as this is a worthwhile, real-world research area where results would be important, if only used descriptively.

Table 7.2 provides means, standard deviations, ranges, skewness, and kurtoses for the DVs. Notice that the means for PSYSXB and PROSB are fairly high,

TABLE 7.2
MANOVA Example Descriptive Means, SDs, Range, Skewness, and Kurtosis

Variable	Mean	SD	Min.	Max.	Skewness	Kurtosis
PSYSXB	4.01	0.75	1.67	5.00	−0.6592	−0.1283
PROSB	4.07	0.81	1.00	5.00	−1.0510	0.9266
CONSB	2.05	0.84	1.00	5.00	0.8899	0.4868
CONSEFFB	3.51	1.15	1.00	5.00	−0.4459	−0.8194

Note: SD = Standard Deviation.

TABLE 7.3
Test-Retest Correlations for PSYSX ($N = 527$)

	Pearson Correlation Coefficients, Prob > |r| under H0: Rho = 0	
	PSYSXA	*PSYSXB*
PSYSXA	1.000	0.660
		<0.0001
PSYSXB	0.660	1.000
	<0.0001	

indicating positive psychosexual functioning and high perceived advantages to using condoms in this sample of women. CONSB has a relatively low mean, and CONSEFFB is somewhere in the middle. Standard deviations are all lower than the means, which provides some reassurance that there is relative homogeneity within groups. Skewness values are within the normal range, except for PROSB, which is slightly negatively skewed, indicating a preponderance of positive responses to the perceived advantages of condom use. Kurtosis values are all within the range of normality.

Correlations

Tables 7.3–7.6 provide the test-retest correlations for the four DVs. Note that the 6-month (A to B) test-retest reliability (correlation) coefficient is acceptable (i.e., 0.66) for psychosexual functioning (see Table 7.3).

In Table 7.4, we see that similar to what we found for PSYSX, the 6-month test-retest reliability (correlation) coefficient for pros of condom use is reasonable (i.e., $r = 0.60$).

The 6-month test-retest reliability coefficient for the cons of condom use, presented in Table 7.5, is also adequate (i.e., 0.61).

Similar to the other variables' reliability coefficients, CONSEFF shows sufficient test-retest correlation (i.e., 0.62) over 6 months (see Table 7.6).

TABLE 7.4
Test-Retest Correlations for PROS ($N = 527$)

	Pearson Correlation Coefficients, Prob > |r| under H0: Rho = 0	
	PROSA	*PROSB*
PROSA	1.000	0.604
		<0.0001
PROSB	0.604	1.000
	<0.0001	

TABLE 7.5
Test-Retest Correlations for CONS ($N = 527$)

	CONSA	CONSB
Pearson Correlation Coefficients, Prob > |r| under H0: Rho = 0		
CONSA	1.000	0.613
		<0.0001
CONSB	0.613	1.000
	<1.000	

Table 7.7 presents the test-rest reliability (correlation) coefficient for STAGE, the IV. Stage of condom use shows moderate to high test-retest reliability (i.e., 0.67), suggesting fairly stable measurement over six months.

Table 7.8 provides the correlations among the IVs and DV. An examination of the correlations among the variables does not indicate collinearity (i.e., $rs <$ $0.70 - 0.90$).

MANOVA

Table 7.9 gives the macro-level results from the MANOVA. The F-tests for all four MANOVA summary indices are significant, indicating that there is evidence for group differences on a linear combination of the DVs. One minus Wilks's lambda, which is equal to η^2, a multivariate effect size, is moderately large (i.e., 0.24).

ANOVAS

After finding significant macro-level results with MANOVA, we can proceed to conduct follow-up analyses at the micro level. Four ANOVAs are conducted, one for each DV, with results given in Tables 7.10 to 7.13.

From Table 7.10, we see that the F-test for the follow-up ANOVA on the DV, PSYSXB, is not significant, nor is the R^2 value very high (i.e., 0.01). Thus, it appears that psychosocial functioning is not significantly different across the five stages of condom use.

TABLE 7.6
Test-Retest Correlations for CONSEFF ($N = 527$)

	CONSEFFA	CONSEFFB
Pearson Correlation Coefficients, Prob > |r| under H0: Rho = 0		
CONSEFFA	1.000	0.616
		<0.0001
CONSEFFB	0.616	1.000
	<0.0001	

TABLE 7.7

Test-Retest Correlations for STAGE ($N = 527$)

Pearson Correlation Coefficients,
Prob $> |r|$ under H0: Rho $= 0$

	STAGEA	STAGEB
STAGEA	1.000	0.670
		<0.0001
STAGEB	0.670	1.000
	<0.0001	

TABLE 7.8

Correlations Among DVs and IV ($N = 527$)

Pearson Correlation Coefficients, Prob $> |r|$ under H0: Rho $= 0$

	PSYSXB	PROSB	CONSB	CONSEFFB	STAGEA
PSYSXB	1.000	0.058	−0.320	0.239	−.085
		0.1806	<0.0001	<0.0001	0.0499
PROSB	0.058	1.000	−0.169	0.361	0.226
	0.1806		<0.0001	<0.0001	<0.0001
CONSB	−0.320	−0.169	1.000	−0.489	−.293
	<0.0001	<0.0001		<0.0001	<0.0001
CONSEFFB	0.239	0.361	−0.489	1.000	0.383
	<0.0001	<0.0001	<0.0001		<0.0001
STAGEA	−.085	0.226	−.293	0.383	1.000
	0.0499	<0.0001	<0.0001	<0.0001	

TABLE 7.9

Macro-Level Results for MANOVA

MANOVA Test Criteria and F Approximations for
the Hypothesis of No Overall STAGEA Effect

H = Type III SSCP Matrix for STAGEA
E = Error SSCP Matrix

Statistic	Value	F-Value	df Num	Den	Pr > F
Wilks' Lambda	0.76442	9.11	16	1586.2	<0.0001
Pillai's Trace	0.23880	8.29	16	2088	<0.0001
Hotteling-Lawley Trace	0.30396	9.84	16	1032	<0.0001
Roy's GCR	0.28967	37.80	4	522	<0.0001

TABLE 7.10
Micro-Level ANOVA Results for Psychosexual Functioning

Class	Levels	Values
STAGEA	5	1 2 3 4 5
Number of observations		527

Dependent Variable: PSYSXB

Source	df	Sum of Squares	Mean Square	F-Value	Prob > F
Model	4	3.78105	0.94526	1.69	0.1502
Error	522	291.42429	0.55828		
Corrected total	526	295.20534			

Root MSE		0.747184	R-Square	0.012808	
Dependent Mean		4.005655			
Coeff Var		18.65323			

Source	df	Type I SS	Mean Square	F-Value	Prob > F
STAGEA	4	3.78105855	0.94526464	1.69	0.1502

TABLE 7.11
Micro-Level ANOVA Results for Pros of Condom Use

Class	Levels	Values
STAGEA	5	1 2 3 4 5
Number of observations		527

Dependent Variable: PROSB

Source	df	Sum of Squares	Mean Square	F-Value	Prob > F
Model	4	18.41366	4.60341	7.42	<0.0001
Error	522	324.06939	0.62082		
Corrected total	526	342.48305			

Root MSE		0.787923	R-Square	0.053765	
Dependent Mean		4.069667			
Coeff Var		19.36087			

Source	df	Type I SS	Mean Square	F-Value	Prob > F
STAGEA	4	18.41366397	4.60341599	7.42	<0.0001

TABLE 7.12
Micro-Level ANOVA Results for Cons of Condom Use

Class	Levels	Values
STAGEA	5	1 2 3 4 5
Number of observations		527

Dependent Variable: CONSB

Source	df	Sum of Squares	Mean Square	F-Value	Prob > F
Model	4	32.61894	8.15473	12.49	<0.0001
Error	522	340.78617	0.65284		
Corrected total	526	373.40512			

Root MSE		0.807990	R-Square	0.087355	
Dependent Mean		2.051550			
Coeff Var		39.38435			

Source	df	Type I SS	Mean Square	F-Value	Prob > F
STAGEA	4	32.618947	8.154736	12.49	<0.0001

TABLE 7.13
Micro-Level ANOVA Results for Condom Self-Efficacy

Class	Levels	Values
STAGEA	5	1 2 3 4 5
Number of observations		527

Dependent Variable: CONSEFFB

Source	df	Sum of Squares	Mean Square	F-Value	Prob > F
Model	4	107.47610	26.86902	23.78	<0.0001
Error	522	589.72271	1.12973		
Corrected total	526	697.19881			

Root MSE		1.062891	R-Square	0.154154	
Dependent Mean		3.514231			
Coeff Var		30.24533			

Source	df	Type I SS	Mean Square	F-Value	Prob > F
STAGEA	4	107.47610	26.86902	23.78	<0.0001

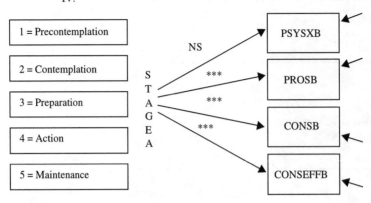

FIG. 7.1. Depiction of Follow-up ANOVA Results in the MANOVA Example with IV = STAGEA and DVs = PSYSXB, PROSB, CONSB, and CONSEFFB NS = No Significant Differences; *** $p < 0.001$.

TABLE 7.14

Micro-Level Tukey Tests for ANOVA on Psychosexual Functioning

Tukey's Studentized Range (HSD) Test for PSYSXB
NOTE: This test controls the Type I experimentwise error rate.

Alpha	0.01
Error Degrees of Freedom	522
Error Mean Square	0.558284
Critical Value of Studentized Range	4.62683

Comparisons significant at the 0.01 level are indicated by ***.

STAGEA	Comparison	Difference Between Means	Simultaneous 99% Confidence Limits		Sig. at 0.01
1	3	0.11408	−0.23939	0.46755	
1	2	0.15376	−0.10867	0.41618	
1	5	0.19680	−0.13853	0.53214	
1	4	0.33101	−0.25068	0.91270	
3	1	−0.11408	−0.46755	0.23939	
3	2	0.03967	−0.29894	0.37829	
3	5	0.08272	−0.31508	0.48052	
3	4	0.21693	−0.40287	0.83673	
2	1	−0.15376	−0.41618	0.10867	
2	3	−0.03967	−0.37829	0.29894	
2	5	0.04305	−0.27659	0.36268	
2	4	0.17725	−0.39553	0.75004	
5	1	−0.19680	−0.53214	0.13853	
5	3	−0.08272	−0.48052	0.31508	
5	2	−0.04305	−0.36268	0.27659	
5	4	0.13421	−0.47543	0.74385	
4	1	−0.33101	−0.91270	0.25068	
4	3	−0.21693	−0.83673	0.40287	
4	2	−0.17725	−0.75004	0.39553	
4	5	−0.13421	−0.74385	0.47543	

TABLE 7.15

Micro-Level Tukey Tests for ANOVA on Pros of Condom Use

Tukey's Studentized Range (HSD) Test for PROSB
NOTE: This test controls the Type I experimentwise error rate.

Alpha	0.01
Error Degrees of Freedom	522
Error Mean Square	0.620823
Critical Value of Studentized Range	4.62683

Comparisons significant at the 0.01 level are indicated by ***.

STAGEA	Comparison	Difference Between Means	Simultaneous 99% Confidence Limits		Sig. at 0.01
5	3	0.26381	−0.15567	0.68330	
5	4	0.33014	−0.31274	0.97302	
5	2	0.40367	0.06660	0.74073	***
5	1	0.57162	0.21801	0.92524	***
3	5	−0.26381	−0.68330	0.15567	
3	4	0.06633	−0.58727	0.71992	
3	2	0.13986	−0.21722	0.49693	
3	1	0.30781	−0.06493	0.68056	
4	5	−0.33014	−0.97302	0.31274	
4	3	−0.06633	−0.71992	0.58727	
4	2	0.07353	−0.53048	0.67754	
4	1	0.24149	−0.37192	0.85489	
2	5	−0.40367	−0.74073	−0.06660	***
2	3	−0.13986	−0.49693	0.21722	
2	4	−0.07353	−0.67754	0.53048	
2	1	0.16796	−0.10878	0.44469	
1	5	−0.57162	−0.92524	−0.21801	***
1	3	−0.30781	−0.68056	0.06493	
1	4	−0.24149	−0.85489	0.37192	
1	2	−0.16796	−0.44469	0.10878	

Table 7.11 reveals that the F-test for the follow-up ANOVA on the DV, PROSB, is significant [$F(4, 522) = 7.42$, $p < 0.0001$], with a small to moderate effect size (i.e., $R^2 = 0.05$). Following the presentation of the ANOVAs, it will be worthwhile to examine Tukey tests between pairs of groups to assess which stages are showing significant differences for PROSB.

Table 7.12 shows that, as with the previous variable, the F-test for the follow-up ANOVA on CONSB is significant [$F(4, 522) = 12.49$, $p < .0001$), with a moderate effect size (i.e., $R^2 = 0.09$). Thus, it will be worth investigating follow-up Tukey tests to assess which stages are showing significant differences in CONSB.

The follow-up ANOVA for CONSEFFB (see Table 7.13) reveals a significant F-test [$F(4, 522) = 23.78$, $p < 0.0001$)], with a large effect size (i.e., $R^2 = 0.15$). We will be interested in determining which stages show significant differences on CONSEFFB when conducting Tukey tests on pairs of means, which we turn to shortly.

TABLE 7.16

Micro-Level Tukey Tests for ANOVA on Cons of Condom Use

Tukey's Studentized Range (HSD) Test for CONSB

NOTE: This test controls the Type I experimentwise error rate.

Alpha	0.01
Error Degrees of Freedom	522
Error Mean Square	0.652847
Critical Value of Studentized Range	4.62683

Comparisons significant at the 0.01 level are indicated by ***.

STAGEA	Comparison	Difference Between Means	Simultaneous 99% Confidence Limits		Sig. at 0.01
1	2	0.14281	−0.14097	0.42659	
1	3	0.27687	−0.10537	0.65911	
1	4	0.58758	−0.04144	1.21661	
1	5	0.72844	0.36581	1.09106	***
2	1	−0.14281	−0.42659	0.14097	
2	3	0.13406	−0.23212	0.50023	
2	4	0.44477	−0.17462	1.06417	
2	5	0.58562	0.23998	0.93127	***
3	1	−0.27687	−0.65911	0.10537	
3	2	−0.13406	−0.50023	0.23212	
3	4	0.31071	−0.35953	0.98096	
3	5	0.45157	0.02140	0.88174	***
4	1	−0.58758	−1.21661	0.04144	
4	2	−0.44477	−1.06417	0.17462	
4	3	−0.31071	−0.98096	0.35953	
4	5	0.14085	−0.51840	0.80011	
5	1	−0.72844	−1.09106	−0.36581	***
5	2	−0.58562	−0.93127	−0.23998	***
5	3	−0.45157	−0.88174	−0.02140	***
5	4	−0.14085	−0.80011	0.51840	

Figure 7.1 depicts the overall ANOVA results with the stages of the categorical IV preceding (by 6 months) the four continuous DVs for this MANOVA example. In the micro-level results that follow, we examine whether there are significant differences across the stages for each of the DVs.

Tukey's Tests of Honestly Significant Differences Between Groups

Tables 7.14-7.17 provide micro-level Tukey tests for each of the DVs. These results show whether there were significant differences between pairs of groups across the five stages of condom use. From Table 7.14, we see that none of the Tukey tests is significant for PSYSXB, consistent with the nonsignificant ANOVA for this DV.

TABLE 7.17
Micro-Level Tukey Tests for ANOVA on Condom Self-Efficacy

Tukey's Studentized Range (HSD) Test for CONSEFFB
NOTE: This test controls the Type I experimentwise error rate.

Alpha	0.01
Error Degrees of Freedom	522
Error Mean Square	1.129737
Critical Value of Studentized Range	4.62683

Comparisons significant at the 0.01 level are indicated by ***.

STAGEA	Comparison	Difference Between Means	Simultaneous 99% Confidence Limits		Sig. at 0.01
5	4	0.4242	−0.4430	1.2914	
5	3	0.7659	0.2000	1.3317	***
5	2	0.8667	0.4120	1.3214	***
5	1	1.3901	0.9131	1.8672	***
4	5	−0.4242	−1.2914	0.4430	
4	3	0.3417	−0.5400	1.2234	
4	2	0.4425	−0.3723	1.2573	
4	1	0.9659	0.1385	1.7934	***
3	5	−0.7659	−1.3317	−0.2000	***
3	4	−0.3417	−1.2234	0.5400	
3	2	0.1008	−0.3809	0.5825	
3	1	0.6243	0.1215	1.1271	***
2	5	−0.8667	−1.3214	−0.4120	***
2	4	−0.4425	−1.2573	0.3723	
2	3	−0.1008	−0.5825	0.3809	
2	1	0.5235	0.1502	0.8968	***
1	5	−1.3901	−1.8672	−0.9131	***
1	4	−0.9659	−1.7934	−0.1385	***
1	3	−0.6243	−1.1271	−0.1215	***
1	2	−0.5235	−0.8968	−0.1502	***

Table 7.15 delineates the Tukey tests conducted on pairs of means for the DV PROSB, showing that individuals in STAGEA 5 (maintaining condom use for 6 months or longer) perceive significantly ($p < 0.01$) more advantages or PROS to using condoms than individuals in either STAGEA 2 (contemplating condom use) or STAGEA 1 (precontemplation, or not even considering condoms).

In Table 7.16, Tukey tests between pairs of groups indicate three significant differences for CONS ($p < 0.01$). Individuals in STAGEA 5 (maintenance) perceive significantly less disadvantages or CONS to using condoms than individuals in either STAGEA 1 (precontemplation), STAGEA 2 (contemplation), or STAGEA 3 (preparation).

Table 7.17 shows that Tukey tests for CONSEFFB reveal significant differences ($p < 0.01$) between six pairs of groups. Individuals in STAGEA 5 (maintenance)

TABLE 7.18

Least-Squares Means for the Four DVs over the Five Stages of the IV

	Least Squares Means			
STAGEA	*PSYSXB LSMEAN*	*PROSB LSMEAN*	*CONSB LSMEAN*	*CONSEFFB LSMEAN*
1	4.12350993	3.86565752	2.27924945	2.97571744
2	3.96975490	4.03361345	2.13643791	3.49918301
3	4.00942857	4.17346939	2.00238095	3.60000000
4	3.79250000	4.10714286	1.69166667	3.94166667
5	3.92670732	4.43728223	1.55081301	4.36585366

Note: For STAGEA, 1 = Precontemplation; 2 = Contemplation; 3 = Preparation; 4 = Action; and 5 = Maintenance

TABLE 7.19

Multiplicity, Background, Central, and Interpretation Themes Applied to MANOVA

Themes	*MANOVA*
Multiplicity themes	+*Theory, hypotheses, and empirical research*
Note: + means	+*Controls*: experimental design
multiplicity of	+*Time points*: Repeated measures
theme pertains	+*Samples*: + groups for IV(s)
	+*Measurements*: +IVs, +DVs
Background themes	*Sample data*: Ideally use random selection and assignment
	Measures: Grouping IV(s) (may use covariate(s), making this MANCOVA), 2+ Continuous DVs
	Assumptions: Normality, linearity, homoscedasticity
	Methods: Inferential with experimental design and assumptions met
Central themes	*Variance*: in DVs
	Covariance: among DVs
	Ratio: Between groups/within groups matrices
Interpretation themes	*Macro*: F-test and summary indices (Wilks's lambda, Hotelling-Lawley trace, GCR, and Pillai's trace),
	ES = cohen's d or η^2
	Micro: Follow-up on DV means and on groups
(Questions to ask)	Do groups differ overall & for each DV?
	Are DVs all needed?
	Low-no correlation between groups of IV(s)?
	Low correlations among DVs?
	Are means significantly different, i.e., high between-group variance?
	Are groups sufficiently homogeneous, i.e., low within-group variance?
	Can design support causal inference?

report significantly greater self-efficacy for using condoms than individuals in either STAGEA 3 (preparation), STAGEA 2 (contemplation), or STAGEA 1 (precontemplation). Further, individuals in STAGEA 1 (precontemplation) show significantly less condom self-efficacy than individuals in STAGEA 2 (contemplation), STAGEA 3 (preparation), and STAGEA 4 (action).

Least-squares means across the five stages of condom use, for each of the four DVs are presented in Table 7.18. For the first DV, there is a decreasing (but nonsignificant) pattern of psychosexual functioning when moving from STAGEA 1 to STAGEA 4, although psychosexual functioning increases slightly in STAGEA 5. With the DV, PROSB, there is generally an increasing trend across the stages, although it dips slightly during the action STAGEA 4. CONSB shows a clear linear decrease in scores when moving from STAGEA 1 to STAGEA 5, suggesting that the disadvantages to using condoms become much less salient the longer an individual uses condoms. Finally, there is a linearly increasing trend in condom self-efficacy as one moves through the stages of condom use from precontemplation (STAGEA 1) to maintenance (STAGEA 5). This indicates that individuals feel much more efficacious about their likelihood of using condoms in the future the longer they actually use condoms.

SUMMARY

A summary of the multiplicity, background, central and interpretation themes for MANOVA is presented in Table 7.19.

REFERENCES

Bock, R. D. (1966). Contributions of multivariate experimental designs to educational research. In Cattell, R. B. (Ed.), *Handbook of multivariate experimental psychology.* Chicago: Rand McNally.

Bock, R. D., & Haggard, E. A. (1968). The use of multivariate analysis of variance in behavioral research. In D. K. Whitla (Ed.), *Handbook of measurement and assessment in behavioral sciences.* Reading, MA: Addison-Wesley.

Cohen, J. (1988). *Statistical power analysis for the behavioral sciences.* San Diego, CA: Academic Press.

Cohen, J. (1992). A power primer. *Psychological Bulletin, 112,* 155–159.

Grimm, L. G., & Yarnold, P. R. (1995). *Reading and understanding multivariate statistics.* Washington, DC: APA.

Harlow, L. L., Quina, K., Morokoff, P. J., Rose, J. S., & Grimley, D. (1993). HIV risk in women: A multifaceted model. *Journal of Applied Biobehavioral Research, 1,* 3–38.

Harris, R. J. (2001). *A primer of multivariate statistics* (3rd ed.). Mahwah, NJ: Lawrence Erlbaum Associates.

Kraemer, H. C., & Thiemann, S. (1987). *How many subjects? Statistical power analysis in research.* Newbury Park, CA: Sage Publications.

Maxwell, S. E., & Delaney, H. D. (2003). *Designing experiments and analyzing data: A model comparison perspective* (2nd ed.). Mahwah, NJ: Lawrence Erlbaum Associates.

Prochaska, J. O., Velicer, W. F., Rossi, J. S., Goldstein, M. G., Marcus, B. H., Rakowski, W., Fiore, C., Harlow, L. L., Redding, C. A., Rosenbloom, D., & Rossi, S. R. (1994). Stages of change and decisional balance for 12 problem behaviors. *Health Psychology, 13*, 39–46.

Tabachnick, B. G., & Fidell, L. S. (2001). *Using multivariate statistics* (4th ed.). Boston: Allyn and Bacon.

Tukey, J. W. (1953). *The problem of multiple comparisons.* Unpublished manuscript, Princeton University (mimeo).

Wilks, S. S. (1932). Certain generalizations in the analysis of variance. *Biometrika, 24*, 471–494.

8

Discriminant Function Analysis

Themes Applied to Discriminant Function Analysis (DFA)

DFA is the first method we discuss that uses a categorical outcome or dependent variable (DV). It is a rigorous multivariate method and shares much in common with multivariate analysis of variance (MANOVA) (Chapter 7), in terms of its mathematics, though the focus for research questions and interpretation may be more similar to multiple regression (MR) (see Chapter 4) and to some extent logistic regression (LR) (see Chapter 9). Interested readers can investigate other descriptions of DFA in several excellent texts (e.g., Grimm, & Yarnold, 1995; Huberty, 1994; Johnson & Wichern, 2002; Tabachnick, & Fidell, 2001). We approach DFA with the same 10 questions we used for other methods thus far.

WHAT IS DFA AND HOW IS IT SIMILAR TO AND DIFFERENT FROM OTHER METHODS?

DFA is a multivariate method that uses several usually continuous independent variables (IVs) and one categorical DV. It is mathematically equivalent to MANOVA in that there are one or more categorical variables on one side and two or more continuous variables on the other side. The main difference is that DFA uses the continuous (discriminating) variables as predictors of the categorical group membership DV. So, the focus in DFA is reversed between "independent" and "dependent" variables compared with MANOVA. DFA can be classified as either a group-difference, or a prediction, statistical analysis. It is mainly used in examining what variables differentiate between groups most clearly. In this sense, the focus is on the groups. However, it is also analogous to a MR analysis except that the dependent or outcome variable is categorical (with several levels or groups) with DFA, instead of continuous (as with MR). Similar to MR, DFA focuses on the weights, often the standardized ones, associated with each of the predictor variables. The variable(s) with the highest standardized discriminant weights are those that will also show the strongest group differences, so that these variables discriminate most clearly among the groups. DFA is also similar to LR except that LR often uses categorical, as well as continuous IVs, and it does not require the traditional general linear model assumptions (i.e., normality, linearity, and homoscedasticity) needed with DFA, MANOVA, MR, and other linear methods. DFA is also similar to canonical correlation (CC) and principal components analysis–factor analysis (PCA-FA) in that all three methods tend to focus on loadings that are correlations between variables and linear combinations or dimensions. We hear more about LR in Chapter 9, CC in Chapter 10, and PCA-FA in Chapter 11.

WHEN IS DFA USED AND WHAT RESEARCH QUESTIONS CAN IT ADDRESS?

DFA is usually used in one of the three ways suggested below:

a. **DFA can be used as a follow-up procedure to a significant MANOVA.** In this case, the DFA would use the continuous DVs from MANOVA as predictors with the groups from MANOVA used as levels of a categorical DV for DFA. The question would be which continuous, discriminating variables were differentiating among the groups most strongly? These would be indicated by a high absolute value for either the standardized discriminant weights, or the discriminant loadings (weights analogous to factor loadings) for those variables. For example, using the reading example mentioned in the last chapter, it would be of interest to know whether reading comprehension or vocabulary was differentiating between the control and treatment groups most strongly. This would provide information about whether the treatment affected reading comprehension or vocabulary or some combination of these.

b. **DFA may be used as a stand-alone prediction analysis** for independent predictor variables that are usually continuous and an outcome variable that has two or more categorical groups. For example, we could predict who would use versus who would not use condoms from several behavioral, interpersonal, and attitudinal predictor variables.

c. **DFA is sometimes used as a classification tool** to assess the degree to which individuals can be correctly classified into groups, based on a number of continuous predictor variables. For example, we could examine the percentage of correct classifications into several diagnostic groups (e.g., depressives, schizophrenics, borderlines) based on several background characteristics and symptoms.

WHAT ARE THE MAIN MULTIPLICITY THEMES FOR DFA?

The multiplicity themes for DFA are very similar to those for MANOVA because the two methods are mathematically the same. Thus, it is important to evaluate multiple theories and previous empirical studies when considering a study using DFA. It is also important to carefully consider multiple continuous predictor variables as well as a relevant categorical outcome variable that has clear categories. Ideally, a researcher should plan to have approximately equal numbers of participants across each of the categories of the DV, although this is not always possible. Using equal category sizes ensures greater robustness of the results. As with most statistical methods, it would be helpful to minimize any redundancy, either in the choice of IVs or in the nature of the categories for the DV. This would help avoid collinearity problems and help ensure clear discrimination among the groups or categories of the DV.

When possible, it is also a good idea to use longitudinal data, possibly collecting both the predictor variables and the DV at an initial time point and again at one or more follow-up time points. This would allow examination of direction of prediction between the IVs and DV to help determine which come first. If a researcher is also able to collect data on multiple samples, this allows an opportunity to investigate cross-validation and the generalizability of one's findings.

WHAT ARE THE MAIN BACKGROUND THEMES APPLIED TO DFA?

Background themes for DFA are very similar to those for MANOVA. We would start by examining a reasonably large ($N \times p$) data matrix that has several (probably continuous) IVs and a categorical DV with two or more groups. When possible, the number of participants in each of the DV groups should be approximately equal. As we did with MANOVA, it would be useful to conduct power analyses to determine the number of participants needed per group to find the expected effect size(s). In the last chapter, we found that if a medium effect size is expected, we would like to have about 68 participants per group to detect our finding with 80% power and alpha $= 0.05$. All the stage groups we have been examining have at least 68 participants except for the action stage in which only 20 or so people (depending on the time point) are involved. This low group size, coupled with the highly uneven sample sizes across all the groups (i.e., $N = 151, 204, 70, 20$, and 82, for STAGEA 1–5, respectively) could serve to lower the power and robustness of a study with these categories.

We also would want to examine descriptive statistics (e.g., means or frequencies, standard deviations, skewness, and kurtosis) as well as correlations among all the variables. The reliability of the variables also should be checked, most likely using either internal consistency or test-retest coefficients. Lastly, we would want to check the assumptions of normality, homoscedasticity, and linearity. As with other methods, a cursory assessment of assumptions could be accomplished by examining skewness, kurtosis, and scatter plots.

WHAT IS THE STATISTICAL MODEL THAT IS TESTED WITH DFA?

With DFA, the main model of interest focuses on linear combinations of the predictor variables, which are usually continuous variables serving as IVs and thus are labeled as Xs for this method:

$$Vi = b1X1 + b2X2 + \cdots + bpXp \tag{8.1}$$

where Vi is a linear combination, b is an (unstandardized) eigenvector weight, X is a predictor IV, and p is the number of predictor IVs.

In DFA, just as with MANOVA, we can form one or more linear combinations, where the number is determined by:

$$\text{number of } Vis = \text{minimum } (p, k - 1), \tag{8.2}$$

where for DFA, p is now the number of independent or predictor variables, and k is the number of groups or levels of the categorical dependent variable. For example, when using an outcome with five categories or groups (e.g., stage of readiness to use condoms) and six predictor variables, we could form four linear combination variables (i.e., the minimum of $[6, 5-1] = 4$). Each of the linear combinations would be orthogonal to each other and would weight the variables slightly differently. Further, not all the linear combinations would be equally effective in differentiating among the groups. We see this more clearly when discussing macro- and micro-assessment later in the chapter.

In contrast to MANOVA that did not focus on these linear combinations, but rather on the means, DFA is very much focused on the weighted combinations, labeled discriminant functions or discriminant scores. Some computer programs also label these as canonical variates.

Just as with MANOVA, for DFA we focus on the ratio of between-group variance over within-group variance matrices: $\mathbf{E}^{-1}\mathbf{H}$, where, again, $\mathbf{E}^{-1}$ represents the inverse of the error or within-group matrix and **H** represents the hypothesis or between-group matrix.

Later we discuss how we evaluate this ratio of matrices at a macro-level and then follow this up with micro-level assessment.

HOW DO CENTRAL THEMES OF VARIANCE, COVARIANCE, AND LINEAR COMBINATIONS APPLY TO DFA?

With DFA, as with MANOVA, we are very interested in the ratio of the variance between groups over the variance within groups. We would like this ratio to be large, indicating that there is a significant relationship between the categorical grouping variable and the best linear combination(s) of the predictor variables. Similar to MR, we are also very interested in the covariances among the predictor variables because they are most likely correlated (i.e., not orthogonal) and DFA takes this into account.

A possible cause of confusion in DFA, or at least a source of complexity, is that we sometimes have to interpret several linear combinations or discriminant functions (i.e., see equation 8.2). A good way to think about this is that DFA allows us to consider several dimensions in which the predictor variables could distinguish among the categories of the grouping variable. This is very similar to examining multiple dimensions or factors in a factor or principal component analysis, methods that we become more familiar with later in Chapter 11. For now, view the possibility of multiple linear combinations as a source of rich grounds for interpreting differences among the groups. There may not be just one way in which the groups differ but multiple ways (i.e., the number of ways is equal to the minimum of $k - 1$ or p as given in equation 8.2).

We also see how the variance of a linear combination, which is an eigenvalue and is labeled a discriminant criterion in DFA, will tell us something about the importance of a discriminant function. This becomes clearer when we discuss interpretation themes, which we turn to in the next section.

WHAT ARE THE MAIN THEMES NEEDED TO INTERPRET DFA RESULTS AT A MACRO-LEVEL?

DFA and MANOVA are mathematically the same and can be assessed with the same macro-level indices (e.g., Wilks's lambda and F-test). However, with DFA, we are much more interested in the linear combinations of variables that are formed with both DFA and MANOVA. So, with DFA, it is worthwhile to describe how these linear combinations or discriminant functions are evaluated. These are evaluated with a single macro-level *F*-test, followed by one or more midlevel *F*-tests, one for each linear combination.

Significance Test

For DFA, just as with MANOVA, we can summarize the variance in the $\mathbf{E}^{-1}\mathbf{H}$ matrix by either of the four macro-summary indices presented previously (see Chapter 7):

    i. Wilks's lambda, and its associated *F*-test;
    ii. The Hotelling–Lawley trace, and its associated *F*-test;
    iii. Pillai's trace, along with its *F*-test; and
    iv. Roy's greatest characteristic root (GCR), and the accompanying *F*-test.

If the overall macro-level *F*-test is significant, this indicates there is significant association between the grouping variable and the linear combinations of predictor variables. We also would want to evaluate a macro-level effect size, just as we did with MANOVA.

Effect Size (ES)

With DFA, as with MANOVA, we can examine eta-squared (i.e., $\eta^2 = 1 - \Lambda$), which indicates how much shared variance there is between the grouping variable and the best linear combination(s) of the predictor variables. We also can use Cohen's (1992) guidelines for small (i.e., 0.02), medium (i.e., 0.13), and large (i.e., 0.26) multivariate effect sizes.

In DFA, we not only want to look at macro-level or big picture results and micro-level or specific findings, we also want to look at *midlevel results* that describe something about the linear combinations, before getting to the specific, variable level weights we will be discussing shortly.

Significance F-Tests

After examining and finding a significant macro-level *F*-test in DFA, we would want to examine the mid-level *F*-tests, where there will be as many of these *F*-tests as there are linear combinations. When the first mid-level *F*-test is significant, this indicates that at least the first linear combination is significantly related to the grouping variable. If a second mid-level *F*-test is significant, this indicates that there is a second linear combination score or discriminant function that significantly differentiates the groups of the categorical outcome variable, and so on until all the *F*-tests have been examined. Notice that the first mid-level *F*-test is actually the same as the macro-level *F*-test. This is because, with DFA, the whole set of linear combinations is examined in the first *F*-test; if it is significant, we conclude that at least the first linear combination is significant, although literally it is all the discriminant functions that are being tested in the first step.

Effect Size

A second point of assessment at the mid-level has to do with the eigenvalues (i.e., discriminant criteria) for each of the linear combinations or discriminant functions. We would like to take note of the size of each eigenvalue, remembering that this tells us about the variance of a discriminant function. The mid-level F-tests inform us about the statistical significance of these eigenvalues or discriminant criteria. We also can form a ratio of discriminant function variance over total variance to find how much of the available discriminatory power is attributed to a specific discriminant function. Thus, we can calculate:

$$\text{index of discriminatory power (IDP)} = \lambda_i / \Sigma\lambda_i, \tag{8.3}$$

where λ_i refers to the ith eigenvalue or discriminant criterion, and $\Sigma\lambda_i$ refers to the sum of all the discriminant criteria. The sum of all the IDP values adds up to 1.0 and thus cannot be interpreted as a proportion of shared variance such as with an ES. We could, however, convert this index to a shared-variance effect size by multiplying each IDP by the macro-level η^2 (i.e., $1 - \Lambda$). I would like to label this new, mid-level effect size-ratio as the "Bowker index" (BI) because a former graduate student, Diane Bowker, first suggested this to me in a multivariate class that I teach (D. Bowker, personal communication, March 22, 1994). Thus,

$$\text{BI}_i = \text{IDP}_i(\eta^2), \tag{8.4}$$

where BI_i indicates the proportion of shared variance between the categorical outcome and the ith specific linear combination of the continuous predictors, IDP_i refers to the index of discriminatory power for a specific ith eigenvalue, and η^2 refers to the macro-level effect size, $1 - \Lambda$. The sum of the BIs will equal the total η^2, with the first BI most likely being much larger than the remaining values:

$$\Sigma\text{BI}_i = \eta^2. \tag{8.5}$$

WHAT ARE THE MAIN THEMES NEEDED TO INTERPRET DFA RESULTS AT A MICRO-LEVEL?

Weights

For each significant discriminant function, we can also examine the weights for each of the predictors. Similar to MR, weights can be unstandardized or standardized, with the latter used for interpreting the relative contribution of each of the continuous variables in separating the groups. In contrast to other methods we have discussed so far, however, there is a third set of weights for DFA. This third set, called discriminant or canonical loadings, is the most interpretable and shows the correlation between a predictor variable and the linear combination or discriminant function. These loadings can be interpreted like part-whole correlations with high absolute values indicating greater discriminatory power. Although significance tests are not usually provided for standardized discriminant weights or loadings, we can interpret them as we would do with correlations with those greater than | 0.30 | being worthwhile to interpret.

Effect Size

Although not always calculated, we could square discriminant loadings (or standardized discriminant weights) to get the proportion of shared variance between a variable and the underlying linear combination (i.e., discriminant function). These effect sizes could be interpreted with univariate, micro-level guidelines of 0.01, 0.06, and 0.13 for small, medium, and large ESs, respectively (Cohen, 1992).

WHAT ARE SOME OTHER CONSIDERATIONS OR NEXT STEPS AFTER APPLYING DFA?

When conducting a DFA, similar to most analyses, we can make only causal inferences to the extent that participants were randomly assigned to groups in which the categorical variable was manipulated. This situation is highly unlikely with DFA because we often are just measuring intact groups. Thus, interpretation should be cautious.

When possible, it would be helpful to follow up a DFA with an experimental design that explored the nature of the relationships between the grouping and discriminating variables in a more rigorous way.

Another consideration is whether sufficient controls were included in a DFA study. Controls could take the form of statistical covariates that may be related to the outcome but that are not the main focus of the study. Another control is to include longitudinal data that provide some evidence of the temporal ordering of the variables.

Still another consideration is whether the results could be affected by the particular sample that is selected. For example, in the data set that we have been analyzing, there are only women from a small New England community. Results could be replicated in a sample of men and also in samples of both men and women from different geographic areas.

Finally, measures should be evaluated about their psychometric integrity. Were the items adequately tapping the construct under study? Was the reliability sufficiently large (e.g., at least 0.70)? If the answer is "no" to either question, more attention should be addressed to improving the nature of the measures in a future study.

WHAT IS AN EXAMPLE OF APPLYING DFA TO A RESEARCH QUESTION?

For DFA, we present two examples. The first is a follow-up to a significant MANOVA, where we build on the MANOVA findings from the previous chapter. In this follow-up form, DFA uses the four continuous variables (i.e., PROSB, pros of condom use; CONSB, cons of condom use; CONSEFFB, self-efficacy for condom use; and PSYSXB, psychosexual functioning) measured at time 2 or B as IVs, with the categorical STAGEA of condom use variable as an outcome. Although this does not make intuitive sense to have predictors at time 2 and an outcome at time 1, we will ignore the timing because we are not attributing causal direction. Instead, we are simply following up a significant MANOVA to assess which continuous variables most likely are showing the largest (i.e., discriminating) group differences. Remember that these discriminating variables will be the ones that have the largest standardized weights or discriminant loadings.

We also present a second, stand-alone DFA, where four continuous predictors are examined at the initial (A) time point, and the categorical outcome, STAGEB of condom use, is examined 6 months later (at time 2 or B). Similar to the examples from previous chapters, the current DFA analyses are based on both the transtheoretical model (e.g., Prochaska et al., 1994) and the multifaceted model of HIV risk (Harlow et al., 1993).

Results are provided in Tables 8.1 to 8.17 for several sets of analyses: DFA follow-up after a significant MANOVA including classification assessment, descriptive statistics for stand-alone DFA with $t1$ predictor variables and a $t2$ categorical variable, correlations for stand-alone DFA, and DFA stand-alone analysis that also examines classification information. Note that we do not repeat the descriptive statistics for the initial DFA follow-up analyses because we already examined these in the MANOVA chapter.

DFA Follow-up Results

In Table 8.1, notice that the macro-level DFA findings are identical to what we found when conducting a MANOVA on these same data. This is expected because the two methods examine the same variables and relationships among the variables at this omnibus level. Thus, we see again that the macro-level F-test, $F(16, 1586) = 9.11$, $p < 0.0001$, Wilks's lambda is 0.76442, and we could calculate η^2 as

TABLE 8.1
Macro-Level Results for the Follow-up DFA

The DISCRIMINANT Procedure

Observations	527	DF Total	526
Variables	4	DF Within Classes	522
Classes	5	DF Between Classes	4

Class Level Information

STAGEA	Freq.	Weight	Proportion	Prior Prob.
1 = Precontemplation	151	151.0000	0.286528	0.200000
2 = Contemplation	204	204.0000	0.387097	0.200000
3 = Preparation	70	70.0000	0.132827	0.200000
4 = Action	20	20.0000	0.037951	0.200000
5 = Maintenance	82	82.0000	0.155598	0.200000

Multivariate Statistics and F Approximations for Follow-up DFA

Statistic	Value	F- Value	df Num.	df Den.	Pr. > F
Wilks' Lambda	0.76442	9.11	16	1586.2	<0.0001
Pillai's Trace	0.23880	8.29	16	2088	<0.0001
Hotelling-Lawley Trace	0.30396	9.84	16	1032	<0.0001
Roy's GCR	0.28967	37.80	4	522	<0.0001

$1 - \Lambda = 0.23558 \approx 0.24$. As before, this indicates a moderately high effect size showing that 24% of the variance in the categorical grouping variable is shared with the best linear combination(s) of the continuous (discriminating) variables. We would now want to examine the magnitude and significance of the discriminant criteria (i.e., eigenvalues) and their associated midlevel F-tests. Subsequently, we will examine micro-level information only for those discriminant functions that are significant.

At the midlevel (see Table 8.2) note that there are four [i.e., min $(k - 1, p)$] linear combinations or discriminant functions formed, generating four eigenvalues (i.e., discriminant criteria), one for each function. The first eigenvalue is much larger than the remaining three, suggesting that most of the shared variance between the categorical and continuous variables involves only the first discriminant function. In the far right column of the middle of Table 8.2, I calculated the BI values (see equation 8.5). These values sum to the total η^2 value (i.e., 0.24), so that the individual BI values can be seen as midlevel effect sizes for the discriminant functions. Only the first BI value is noteworthy, indicating a moderately large multivariate ES for the first discriminant function. The importance of only one linear combination is also evident when examining the F-tests for each discriminant function. The first F-test is significant, indicating that at least the first discriminant function is significant. Notice, however, that none of the other discriminant functions has a

TABLE 8.2
Mid-Level Results for the Follow-up DFA

(Canonical) Discriminant Analysis for Follow-up DFA

v	Canonical [discriminant] Correlation	Adj. Canonical [discriminant] Correlation	Approximate Standard Error	Squared Canonical [discriminant] Correlation
1	0.473931	0.464792	0.033809	0.224611
2	0.093495	.	0.043221	0.008741
3	0.071264	.	0.043381	0.005079
4	0.019277	.	0.043586	0.000372

[Eigenvalues of Inv(E) *H] = CanRsq/(1-CanRsq)

v	Eigenvalue	Proportion = IDP values	Cumulative	BI
1	0.289675	0.952972	0.952972	0.2245
2	0.008818	0.029009	0.981981	0.0068
3	0.005105	0.016794	0.998775	0.0040
4	0.000372	0.001224	0.999999	0.003
				Σ(BI) ≈ 0.24

v	Likelihood Ratio	Approximate F-Value	Num. df	Den. df	Pr. > F
1	0.76442373	9.11	16	1586.2	<0.0001
2	0.98585807	0.83	9	1265.7	0.5927
3	0.99455177	0.71	4	1042	0.5834
4	0.99962838	0.19	1	522	0.6597

significant associated *F*-test. Thus, we would want to interpret the discriminant weights only for the first discriminant function.

Table 8.3 gives the pooled within canonical structure, which yields the discriminant loadings that are the most interpretable weights to examine in DFA. These loadings can be interpreted as correlations between the specific discriminating variable (on the independent or left side) and the overall linear combination (i.e., discriminant function). Because significance tests are not readily available for these loadings, we use a guideline that loadings, like correlations, can be interpreted

TABLE 8.3
Micro-Level Discriminant Loadings for the Follow-up DFA

Pooled Within Canonical Structure [i.e., Discriminant Loadings] for Follow-up DFA

Variable	v1	v2	v3	v4
PSYSXB	−0.178186	−0.563405	0.394348	0.703785
PROSB	0.428439	−0.336544	0.710217	−0.445836
CONSB	−0.559740	0.702903	0.334776	−0.283801
CONSEFFB	0.791755	0.078818	0.314175	0.517886

TABLE 8.4
Micro-Level Unstandardized Discriminant Weights for the Follow-up DFA

| | Raw Canonical Coefficients [i.e., Unstandardized Discriminant Weights] | | | |
Variable	v1	v2	v3	v4
PSYSXB	−0.762850	−0.603109	0.698234	0.834467
PROSB	0.263050	−0.533358	0.850278	−0.836804
CONSB	−0.541600	0.970289	0.878886	0.147165
CONSEFFB	0.671011	0.639986	0.241716	0.546780

as meaningful when greater than or equal to | 0.30 |. With this criterion, three of the four variables have loadings on the first discriminant function (i.e., V1) that are worth examining. As with the follow-up ANOVAs in the MANOVA chapter, the continuous variable that shows the biggest differences across the STAGE groups is also the variable (i.e., condom self-efficacy B) that has the highest discriminant loading (i.e., 0.79). The next highest loading is associated with the cons (i.e., −0.56), followed by the pros of condom use (i.e., 0.43). Thus, this first discriminant function is largely focused on condom self-efficacy and, to a lesser degree, the pros and cons of condom use. [Note that we do not have to examine loadings for the other three functions (i.e., V2 to V4) as these were not significant in the midlevel assessment.] If we checked back to the MANOVA chapter, we would realize that these same three variables (CONSEFFB, CONSB, and PROSB) were the measures that showed significant differences across the stages of condom use, showing a link between high (absolute value) discriminant loadings and group differences.

Given the unstandardized discriminant weights (i.e., raw canonical coefficients) in Table 8.4, we could form a discriminant function score from the first column:

$$V_1 = -0.76(\text{PSYSXB}) + 0.26(\text{PROSB}) - 0.54(\text{CONSB}) + 0.67(\text{CONSEFFB}).$$

This could be useful in a future prediction study if we knew the scores for the four continuous variables. Remember, however, that we cannot interpret the importance or magnitude of the relationship between a continuous variable and its discriminant function with *unstandardized* weights. This is best handled with discriminant loadings (see above) or, when not available, with standardized discriminant weights.

It is also sometimes informative to examine the group centroids (see Table 8.5), which are listed as the class means of the canonical variables (i.e., discriminant functions). These are simply the means of the V_i scores for each of the five STAGEA groups. For the first discriminant function (labeled as V1 in Table 8.5), which is the only function we would want to interpret given the pattern of significance, there is more separation between the stages than with the other three discriminant functions. This is because the analyses revealed that the second, third, and fourth discriminant functions were not significantly separating the

TABLE 8.5
Group Centroids for the Follow-up DFA Discriminant Functions

Class Means (i.e., Group Centroids) on Canonical Variables (i.e., Discriminant Functions)

STAGEA	v1	v2	v3	v4
1 = Precontemplation	−0.628	−0.086	−0.021	0.008
2 = Contemplation	−0.038	0.114	0.015	0.004
3 = Preparation	0.109	−0.050	0.068	−0.044
4 = Action	0.654	0.033	−0.329	−0.028
5 = Maintenance	0.999	−0.089	0.023	0.018

groups. Later in the stand-alone example of DFA, we present a graph of the class means or centroids for the first two canonical variates, in which, similar to this example, only the first one is significant.

It is sometimes useful to examine the pattern of predicted to actual group (i.e., STAGE) designation. In Table 8.6, participants are numbered from 1 to N, although only the first seven cases are presented here to conserve space. Both the actual and predicted STAGE classifications are given, and when these are disparate it is indicated by an asterisk. We can see that there is considerable misclassification (i.e., 5 of the first 7 cases), although we know that classification is at least significantly greater than chance because the F-test associated with Wilks's lambda was significant.

Next, we examine the percentages of correct classification for each stage and also overall presented along the diagonal of the classification table. These provide the percentage of correct classification for each stage, which ideally should be greater than (prior) chance (i.e., $1/5 = 0.20$ or 20%: see bottom values of 0.20).

We can see from the classification grid in Table 8.7 that the discriminant functions were reasonably accurate in classifying individuals into Stages 1, 4, and 5

TABLE 8.6
Individual Classification Results for the Follow-up DFA

Posterior Probability of Membership in STAGEA (for Follow-up DFA)

Obs.	Classified from STAGEA	into STAGEA	1	2	3	4	5
1	1	5 *	0.1227	0.2022	0.2188	0.2036	0.2528
2	5	4 *	0.0616	0.1548	0.1575	0.3835	0.2426
3	1	5 *	0.1067	0.1880	0.2432	0.1600	0.3021
4	2	4 *	0.1290	0.1798	0.1976	0.2900	0.2036
5	5	5	0.1240	0.1934	0.2279	0.2146	0.2401
6	3	1 *	0.2726	0.2525	0.2564	0.1146	0.1038
7	1	1	0.2797	0.2490	0.2253	0.1508	0.0952
...							

* Misclassified observation

TABLE 8.7

Classification Table for Actual and Predicted Stages in the Follow-up DFA

# of Observations and % Classified into STAGEA (for Follow-up DFA)

From STAGEA	1	2	3	4	5	Total
1	84	20	18	11	18	151
	55.63	13.25	11.92	7.28	11.92	100%
2	70	27	31	35	41	204
	34.31	13.24	15.20	17.16	20.10	100%
3	23	13	10	9	15	70
	32.86	18.57	14.29	12.86	21.43	100%
4	2	1	1	9	7	20
	10.00	5.00	5.00	45.00	35.00	100%
5	4	4	8	21	45	82
	4.88	4.88	9.76	25.61	54.88	100%
Total	183	65	68	85	126	527
	34.72	12.33	12.90	16.13	23.91	100%
Priors	0.2	0.2	0.2	0.2	0.2	

Error Count Estimates for STAGEA (for Follow-up DFA)

	1	2	3	4	5	Total
Rate	0.4437	0.8676	0.8571	0.5500	0.4512	0.6339
Priors	0.2000	0.2000	0.2000	0.2000	0.2000	

(i.e., 56%, 45%, and 55%, correct classification for these respective stages). The contemplation and action stages show much less accuracy, in fact less than chance (i.e., $< 0.20\%$). The overall percentage of correct classification is found by subtracting the proportion of total error count estimates from 1 and multiplying by 100. Thus, the current discriminant function resulted in 37% correct classification into STAGES, which is greater than a 20% chance classification.

We now turn to an example of a stand-alone DFA with the continuous variables (i.e., psychosexual functioning, pros of condom use, cons of condom use, and condom self-efficacy) at time 1 serving as predictors or discriminating variables, and the stage of condom use, measured 6 months later, serving as the categorical outcome. The interpretation of results is similar to the follow-up form of DFA, although the focus is now more on a predictive model than a follow-up to a group-difference model.

Descriptive Statistics for Stand-Alone DFA

Tables 8.8 and 8.9 provide descriptive statistics for the stand-alone DFA, which uses the same four IVs at time A (i.e., PSYSXA, PROSA, CONSA, and

TABLE 8.8
Descriptive Frequencies for Stand-Alone DFA Example

STAGEB	Freq.	%	Cumulative Frequency	Cumulative Percent
1 = Precontemplation	154	29.22	154	29.22
2 = Contemplation	185	35.10	339	64.33
3 = Preparation	79	14.99	418	79.32
4 = Action	22	4.17	440	83.49
5 = Maintenance	87	16.51	527	100.00

CONSEFFA), and a categorical outcome, STAGEB, measured 6 months later. Frequencies (see Table 8.8) for the stages of condom use B are similar to those from time A, 6 months earlier (see MANOVA Chapter). At both time points, the largest proportion of individuals is at the contemplation stage, followed by those in precontemplation, maintenance, preparation, and the smallest proportion occurring in the action stage. Notice that the means (see Table 8.9) for psychosexual functioning and the pros of condom use are relatively large at this initial time point, similar to what we found for these same variables when measured 6 months later in the MANOVA example from the last chapter. Likewise, the mean for the cons of condom use is relatively low, with the mean for condom self-efficacy falling somewhere in between. Thus, this sample of 527 women at risk for HIV are responding fairly consistently, at least when viewed as a group, over a 6-month period.

Correlations for Stand-Alone DFA

Table 8.10 presents correlations among the variables used in the stand-alone DFA. Correlations among the variables appear reasonable, with none of them even coming close to collinearity levels (i.e., all correlations are $< |0.70|$).

Stand-Alone DFA Results

Even though we are examining different time points for the variables than with the initial DFA, we still find a significant macro-level relationship. The F-test associated with Wilks's lambda is significant ($F = 13.52$, $p < .0001$ in

TABLE 8.9
Descriptive Means, SDs, Range, Skewness, and Kurtosis for Stand-Alone DFA

Variable	Mean	S.D.	Min.	Max.	Skewness	Kurtosis
PSYSXA	3.99	0.76	1.00	5.00	−0.854	0.794
PROSA	3.86	0.95	1.00	5.00	−1.006	0.588
CONSA	2.14	0.90	1.00	5.00	0.710	0.078
CONSEFFA	3.29	1.30	1.00	5.00	−0.306	−1.189

TABLE 8.10
Pearson Correlation Coefficients ($N = 527$) Prob $> |r|$ under H0: Rho $= 0$

	PSYSXA	PROSA	CONSA	CONSEFFA	STAGEB
PSYSXA	1.0000	−0.0189	−0.2240	0.0862	−0.1564
		0.6660	<0.0001	0.0477	0.0003
PROSA	−0.0189	1.0000	−0.0634	0.3150	0.2557
	0.6636		0.1456	<0.0001	<0.0001
CONSA	−0.2240	−0.0634	1.0000	−0.4020	−0.2458
	<0.0001	0.1456		<0.0001	<0.0001
CONSEFFA	0.0862	0.3150	−0.4020	1.0000	0.4840
	0.0477	<0.0001	<0.0001		<0.0001
STAGEB	−0.1564	0.2557	−0.2458	0.4840	1.0000
	0.0003	<0.0001	<0.0001	<0.0001	

Table 8.11), with η^2 equal to 0.32, indicating a large multivariate ES. We would now want to examine which of the individual discriminant functions had significant discriminant criteria or eigenvalues.

Similar to the MANOVA example, there are four discriminant functions, each with their respective eigenvalues and significance tests (see Table 8.12). From the macro-level results presented here, we can see that only the first discriminant

TABLE 8.11
Macro-Level Results for Stand-Alone DFA

The DISCRIM Procedure for the Stand-Alone DFA

Observations	527	DF Total	526
Variables	4	DF Within Classes	522
Classes	5	DF Between Classes	4

Class Level Information

STAGEA	Freq.	Weight	Proportion	Prior Prob.
1 = Precontemplation	154	154.000	0.292	0.200
2 = Contemplation	185	185.000	0.351	0.200
3 = Preparation	79	79.000	0.150	0.200
4 = Action	22	22.000	0.042	0.200
5 = Maintenance	87	87.000	0.165	0.200

Multivariate Statistics and F Approximations (for the Stand-Alone DFA)

Statistics	Value	F-Value	df Num.	df Den.	Pr. > F
Wilks' Lambda	0.67668	13.52	16	1586.2	<0.0001
Pillai's Trace	0.33205	11.81	16	2088	<0.0001
Hotelling-Lawley Trace	0.46494	15.05	16	1032	<0.0001
Roy's GCR	0.43577	56.87	4	522	<0.0001

TABLE 8.12
Mid-Level Results for Stand-Alone DFA

Canonical Discriminant Analysis (for Stand-Alone DFA)

v	Canonical [discriminant] Correlation	Adj. Canonical [discriminant] Correlation	Approximate Standard Error	Squared Canonical [discriminant] Correlation
1	0.550920	0.543905	0.030368	0.303513
2	0.156317	0.131127	0.042537	0.024435
3	0.063770	.	0.043425	0.004067
4	0.005953	.	0.043601	0.000035

[Eigenvalues of Inv (E)*H] / = CanRsq/(1 − CanRsq)

v	Eigenvalues = Discriminant Criteria	Proportion = IDPs	Cumulative	Bowker Index
1	0.4358	0.9373	0.9373	0.3030
2	0.0250	0.0539	0.9911	0.0174
3	0.0041	0.0088	0.9999	0.0028
4	0.0000	0.0000	1.0000	0.0000
				$\sum(BI) \approx$ 0.32

	Likelihood Ratio	Approximate F Value	Num DF	Den DF	Pr > F
1	0.67668094	13.52	16	1586.2	<0.0001
2	0.97156341	1.68	9	1265.7	0.0897
3	0.99589808	0.54	4	1042	0.7094
4	0.99996457	0.02	1	522	0.8919

Test of H0: The canonical correlations in the current row and all that follow are zero (for Stand-alone DFA)

function is significant (see the likelihood ratio and F tests in Table 8.12), though the second one approached significance. Consistent with this result, the first eigenvalue is capturing the bulk of the available variance, with the remaining ones being fairly small. The predominance of the first discriminant function is also evident by its large ES (see BI = 0.30), whereas the ESs for the remaining functions are trivial. Notice also that the first F-test is actually the same as the macro-level test we saw initially. This is because it includes information on all of the eigenvalues, although it is interpreted as providing information on just the first discriminant function. We would now want to examine the weights for this first function.

Table 8.13 presents the micro-level results for the stand-alone DFA. As in the previous example, the variable with the highest discriminant loading (i.e., see pooled within canonical structure) is CONSEFFA, which correlates 0.84 with the first discriminant function. In contrast to the findings with the follow-up

TABLE 8.13
Micro-Level Discriminant Loadings for the Stand-Alone DFA

Pooled Within Canonical Structure [i.e., Discriminant Loadings] for Stand-alone DFA

Variable	V1	V2	V3	V4
PSYSXA	−0.267171	0.544737	0.646691	−0.462245
PROSA	0.424869	−0.647438	0.519540	−0.361094
CONSA	−0.380507	−0.416079	0.313287	0.764163
CONSEFFA	0.836638	0.425562	0.336664	0.074771

DFA, here PROSA has the next highest loading (i.e., 0.42), followed by CONS (i.e., −0.38). As before, PSYSXA does not contribute very much to this discriminant function (i.e., the loading is < | 0.30 |). These findings would tell us that the best predictor of STAGE at time 2 is an individual's level of condom self-efficacy 6 months earlier. Knowing both the perceived pros and cons of condom use would also contribute to the prediction of stage of condom use 6 months later. In both the follow-up and stand-alone DFA, knowing an individual's level of psychosexual functioning does not help in predicting which stage of condom use the person will be in after six months.

Figure 8.1 depicts the stand-alone DFA results with loadings attached to each predictor for the first discriminant function, V1.

Table 8.14 presents the unstandardized discriminant weights for all four discriminant functions (i.e., V1 to V4), although only the first column of weights should

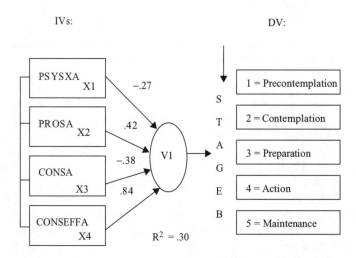

FIG. 8.1. DFA with 4 IVs and 1 DV showing significant R^2 (= 0.30) shared variance, $F(16, 1586) = 13.52$, $p < 0.0001$, with discriminant loadings for 1st function (V1).

TABLE 8.14
Micro-Level Unstandardized Results

	Raw Canonical Coefficients [i.e., Unstandardized Discriminant Weights]			
Variable	V1	V2	V3	V4
PSYSXA	−0.66242430	0.59127098	0.99074467	−0.41408549
PROSA	0.28684962	−0.84359422	0.46624882	−0.50764419
CONSA	−0.29064190	−0.16210037	0.71128384	0.97205961
CONSEFFA	0.69161979	0.41196589	0.26697501	0.45924274

be used because only V1 was significant at the midlevel. If we were interested, we could create a discriminant score for the first function by applying the raw (unstandardized) discriminant weights to the individual variables:

$$V_1 = -0.66\,(\text{PSYSXB}) + 0.29\,(\text{PROSB}) - 0.29\,(\text{CONSB}) + 0.69\,(\text{CONSEFFB}).$$

Table 8.15 gives the group centroids for the four discriminant functions. As with the other results, we would interpret those just for the only significant (first) function. Notice that the function means for V1 are more spread apart than those for the other (nonsignificant) functions (i.e., V2 to V4). This is consistent with the F-test results that showed that only the first function significantly discriminated across the stage groups.

Figure 8.2 visually depicts the discriminating power of the first function by comparing the group centroids for the first discriminant function, V1, with those for the second discriminant function, V2. Notice that the bars representing the centroids for V1 are more spread apart than those for V2.

Table 8.16 presents the individual classification results (labeled: posterior probability of membership into stageB from the stand-alone DFA) for the first seven participants. This lists the stages of condom use from which they started, the stages at which the DFA predicted them, and the probabilities of being classified into each of the five stages. As we did with the follow-up DFA, we can scan the first few columns to see how well the first discriminant function did in classifying individuals

TABLE 8.15
Group Centroids for Stand-Alone DFA Discriminant Functions

	Class Means [i.e., Group Centroids] on Discriminant Functions for Stand-alone DFA			
STAGEB	V1	V2	V3	V4
1 = Precontemplation	−0.763	0.126	−0.027	−0.003
2 = Contemplation	−0.130	−0.089	0.033	0.007
3 = Preparation	0.401	−0.264	−0.069	−0.007
4 = Action	0.372	0.006	0.252	−0.016
5 = Maintenance	1.169	0.206	−0.023	0.001

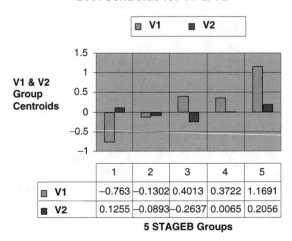

DFA Centroids for V1 & V2

| □ V1 | ■ V2 |

V1 & V2 Group Centroids

	1	2	3	4	5
□ V1	−0.763	−0.1302	0.4013	0.3722	1.1691
■ V2	0.1255	−0.0893	−0.2637	0.0065	0.2056

5 STAGEB Groups

FIG. 8.2. Plot of group centroids for first two discriminant functions.

into the correct stage group. We can see by the number of asterisks, indicating an incorrect classification, that there are many individuals who were not correctly classified into their initial stage category.

Table 8.17 provides the summary classification table for the stand-alone DFA. The stage with the highest percentage of correct classification is maintenance (i.e., 68% of the individuals who were initially listed as in Stage 5 were subsequently classified as Stage 5 based on the discriminant function results). Stage 1 (precontemplation) also fares well with 56% correct classification. In contrast to the DFA

TABLE 8.16
Individual Classification Results for Stand-Alone DFA

Posterior Probability of Membership in STAGEB (for Stand-alone DFA)

Obs.	Classified from STAGEB	into STAGEB	1	2	3	4	5
1	1	1	0.6894	0.1851	0.0564	0.0558	0.0132
2	5	5	0.0140	0.0698	0.2238	0.1389	0.5535
3	1	4 *	0.1395	0.2201	0.1671	0.3464	0.1269
4	2	3 *	0.1165	0.2194	0.3226	0.1744	0.1671
5	1	5 *	0.1056	0.1854	0.2256	0.2245	0.2589
6	2	3 *	0.0670	0.1787	0.2804	0.2515	0.2223
7	1	1	0.4653	0.2755	0.1137	0.1314	0.0141
...							

* Misclassified observation

TABLE 8.17

Classification Table for Actual and Predicted Stages in Stand-Alone DFA

# of Observations and % Classified into STAGEB
Classification Summary for Stand-Alone DFA
Number of Observations and Percent Classified into STAGEB

From STAGEB	1	2	3	4	5	Total
1	86	13	15	27	13	154
	55.84	8.44	9.74	17.53	8.44	100%
2	67	26	29	28	35	185
	36.22	14.05	15.68	15.14	18.92	100%
3	12	8	23	11	25	79
	15.19	10.13	29.11	13.92	31.65	100%
4	3	3	4	3	9	22
	13.64	13.64	18.18	13.64	40.91	100%
5	3	1	10	14	59	87
	3.45	1.15	11.49	16.09	67.82	100%
Total	171	51	81	83	141	527
	32.45	9.68	15.37	15.75	26.76	100%
Priors	0.2	0.2	0.2	0.2	0.2	

Error Count Estimates for STAGEB (for Stand-Alone DFA)

	1	2	3	4	5	Total
Rate	0.4416	0.8595	0.7089	0.8636	0.3218	0.6391
Priors	0.2000	0.2000	0.2000	0.2000	0.2000	

results with the follow-up to the MANOVA example from the previous chapter, individuals in the preparation stage were classified better than chance (i.e., 29% is > 20%). However, the action stage did not do well at all for the current analysis, nor did contemplation, both of which had only 14% correct classification. Thus, if an individual started out in either of these stages there would be only a chance possibility of them being correctly classified into their original stage for both action and contemplation.

From the error count estimates at the bottom of Table 8.17 we see that overall, there was 36% correct classification (i.e., 100 − 64) for this discriminant function predicting membership in STAGEB. This is very similar to what we found earlier (i.e., 37%) with STAGEA in the follow-up DFA results. Thus, we can conclude that the discriminant function did reasonably well in predicting stage of condom use 6 months later, although the variable psychosexual functioning did not contribute very much and probably could be dropped from future research.

TABLE 8.18
Multiplicity, Background, Central, and Interpretation Themes Applied to DFA

Themes	Discriminant Function Analysis
Multiplicity themes Note: + means multiplicity of theme pertains	+*Theory, hypotheses and empirical research* +*Controls*: Experimental design, covariates, select sample +*Time Points*: IVs and/or DV +*Samples*: + DV Groups, Cross validate if possible +*Measurements*: +IVs, +Groups for DV(s)
Background themes	*Sample Data*: Random selection (and assignment) *Measures*: Grouping DV, [Continuous covariate(s),] Multiple continuous IVs *Assumptions*: Normality, linearity, homoscedasticity *Methods*: Inferential with assumptions met
Central themes	*Variance*: in DV shared by discriminant function(s) *Covariance*: between DV and IVs and among IVs *Ratio*: Between groups/within groups variance matrices
Interpretation themes (Questions to ask)	*Macro*: Omnibus χ^2 or F-test, ES $= \eta^2$ *Mid*: F-tests for each eigenvalue (discriminant criteria), and IDP and BI for each discriminant function; and % of correct classification *Micro:* Discriminant weights (standardized or loadings) Do IVs discriminate among DV groups? Are all variables reliable & needed? Low correlations among IVs (i.e., no collinearity)? Significant η^2 or shared variance between IVs and DV? Correct classification into DV groups by set of IVs? Which IVs significantly discriminate among DV groups? Assumptions met? Can design support causal inference?

SUMMARY

A summary of the multiplicity, background, central, and interpretation themes for DFA is presented in Table 8.18.

REFERENCES

Cohen, J. (1992). A power primer. *Psychological Bulletin, 112*, 155–159.
Grimm, L. G., & Yarnold, P. R. (1995). *Reading and understanding multivariate statistics.* Washington, DC: APA.
Harlow, L. L., Quina, K., Morokoff, P. J., Rose, J. S., & Grimley, D. (1993). HIV risk in women: A multifaceted model. *Journal of Applied Biobehavioral Research, 1*, 3–38.
Huberty, C. (1994). *Applied discriminant analyses.* New York: Wiley & Sons.

Johnson, R. A., & Wichern, D. W. (2002). *Applied multivariate statistical analysis* (5th ed.). Englewood Cliffs, NJ: Prentice Hall.

Prochaska, J. O., Velicer, W. F., Rossi, J. S., Goldstein, M. G., Marcus, B. H., Rakowski, W., Fiore, C., Harlow, L. L., Redding, C. A., Rosenbloom, D., & Rossi, S. R. (1994). Stages of change and decisional balance for 12 problem behaviors. *Health Psychology, 13*, 39–46.

Tabachnick, B. G., & Fidell, L. S. (2001). *Using multivariate statistics* (4th ed.) (Chapter 11: pp. 456–516). Boston: Allyn and Bacon.

9

Logistic Regression

Themes Applied to Logistic Regression (LR)

LR is a multivariate prediction method that is most likely to use all or some categorical predictors to explain a categorical, usually dichotomous, outcome. As we will see, it bears similarities and differences to other prediction methods such as multiple regression (MR) and discriminant function anlalysis (DFA) (see Chapters 4 and 8, respectively). Several excellent sources can be consulted regarding logistic regression. Hosmer and Lemeshow (1989) have written what is commonly believed to be the definitive text on LR. Other well-written manuscripts explain the essentials of LR in easy to understand language (e.g., Menard, 1995; Rose, Chassin, Presson & Sherman, 2000; Tabachnick & Fidell [Ch. 12], 2001; Wright, 1995). We now turn to a delineation of how the set of 10 questions and themes pertain to the method of LR.

WHAT IS LR AND HOW IS IT SIMILAR TO AND DIFFERENT FROM OTHER METHODS?

LR is a multivariate method that allows several independent variables (IVs), either categorical or continuous, and a categorical dependent variable (DV). The goal is to assess the likelihood of falling into one of the DV categories, given a set of predictor IVs. Similar to MR, LR allows multiple IVs and a single DV. A distinction, however, is that in MR the outcome is continuous, whereas with LR the outcome is categorical. LR is also similar to DFA in that they both allow multiple predictor IVs and a single categorical DV. LR and DFA differ in the nature of their assumptions, goals, and their output. Traditional assumptions of linearity, homoscedasticity, and normality are usually required for DFA. LR, in contrast, does not require these assumptions, and outcome categories must be exclusive and exhaustive so that each participant must be classified into one, and only one, of the outcome categories. As for objectives and output, DFA usually is focused on the correlational weights for prediction, and the percentage of correct classification of individuals, into group membership. LR is used, particularly in health research, to assess the odds or likelihood of disease given certain characteristics or symptoms. Further, LR usually requires larger samples due to using maximum-likelihood estimation (Wright, 1995).

WHEN IS LR USED AND WHAT RESEARCH QUESTIONS CAN IT ADDRESS?

LR is often used in one of the three ways suggested below:

a. **LR can be used as a prediction method** whenever there are several IVs (either categorical or continuous), and a single dichotomous outcome. This is the simplest and probably the most commonly used form of LR. The goal would be to test whether the set of IVs is significantly related to falling into one of the two outcome categories. For example (Rose et al., 2000), we could predict quitting smoking (1 = successful, 0 = not successful) with predictors such as gender, amount smoked, onset of smoking, and a set of conceptual variables (e.g., smoking environment, smoking beliefs, smoking motives, reasons for quitting, and social reasons for smoking). If the overall set of predictors is significantly related to the outcome of quitting smoking, we could then examine which predictors are most strongly linked with the outcome.

b. **LR also can be used when there are multiple outcome categories** and a set of predictor IVs (either categorical or continuous). The goal, similar to the dichotomous LR, is to assess whether the set of IVs is significantly related to falling into one of the set of outcome categories. Tabachnick and Fidell (2001) present an example to investigate whether a set of demographic and attitudinal IVs can significantly predict group membership into one of three outcome categories (wife employed outside home, satisfied nonemployed housewife, dissatisfied nonemployed housewife).

c. **LR can be used as an exploratory model-building method** in which a number of nested models (models that are subsets of a larger model) are compared to determine the most parsimonious set of predictors needed to adequately predict the likelihood of falling into one of two or more outcome categories. This method is used quite often, but it is the most controversial because it capitalizes on chance variation and often overfits a model to the data. Although it is sometimes advantageous to explore the data to test a variety of models, the problem with this form of LR is that researchers may treat the results with greater generalizability and validity than may be warranted. As with any method, it is always best to cross-validate results on independent samples before generalizing beyond a specific sample and set of variables.

WHAT ARE THE MAIN MULTIPLICITY THEMES FOR LR?

LR is very similar to DFA in the multiplicity themes entailed. As with most multivariate methods, we would like to consider multiple theories and empirical studies before conducting a LR analysis. As with DFA, LR requires the use of a categorical outcome with two or more response categories. We also want to include multiple, reliable IVs to adequately predict membership into one of the outcome categories. Unlike DFA, LR is more likely to include a set of interactions between some of the IVs to enhance prediction. This practice makes it even more important to try and limit collinearity among the IVs because interactions with variables that are already highly related can exacerbate problems with estimation. We also would want to have a large sample to ensure stability and power in our findings. If it were feasible, it would be helpful to collect data from multiple time points to provide some evidence of the direction of causation between IVs and the categorical outcome.

WHAT ARE THE MAIN BACKGROUND THEMES APPLIED TO LR?

Background themes for LR are somewhat similar to those for MR and DFA. We would start by examining a reasonably large ($N \times p$) data matrix that has several IVs and a single (categorical) DV (with two or more groups). To enhance the power of the results, Aldrich and Nelson (1984) recommend a ratio of 50 participants per IV, probably requiring a larger sample size than either MR or DFA. Our LR example (presented later in the chapter) exceeds these guidelines because we use the same sample (i.e., $N = 527$ women at risk for HIV) and variables (i.e., five-category outcome: stage of condom use; and four predictors: psychosexual functioning, pros of condom use, cons of condom use, and self-efficacy of condom use) as with DFA and MR. Thus, our sample appears sufficiently large (i.e., $N > 200$) to use LR.

We also would want to begin a LR analysis by first examining descriptive statistics (e.g., means or frequencies, standard deviations, skewness, and kurtosis), reliability, and correlations among all the variables. Because we are using the same variables as in the stand-alone DFA example presented in Chapter 8, we do not repeat these background analyses in this chapter. Note that the same variables were used in the MR example presented in Chapter 4, although for MR, all the variables were measured at time B, whereas for DFA and LR the IVs are measured at time A and the DV is measured 6 months later at time B.

WHAT IS THE STATISTICAL MODEL THAT IS TESTED WITH LR?

With LR, the model is more complex than it was for DFA or MR, though each of these methods involves some function of weighted predictor variables. In LR, we examine an exponential function for a predicted score, X', but Y is initially modeled as it is with MR:

$$Y = X' + E \qquad (9.1)$$

where Y is a categorical outcome variable, E is prediction error, and X' is a ratio of exponential functions of the linear equation we saw in MR:

$$X' = A + B_1X_1 + B_2X_2 + B_3X_3 + \cdots + B_pX_p, \qquad (9.2)$$

With a dichotomous outcome, Y (where $Y = 1$ or 0), and 4 predictor X variables, we would have:

$$X' = [e^{A+B1X1+B2X2+B3X3+B4X4}]/[1 + e^{A+B1X1+B2X2+B3X3+B4X4}] \qquad (9.3)$$

where X' is a probability value ranging from 0 and 1.

With LR, as with MR, the values for the A (i.e., constant) and B weights are the unstandardized coefficients associated with each predictor variable.

In contrast to MR and DFA, the weights that we usually interpret with LR are called *odds ratios*. These indicate the chance of being in an outcome category given a one-unit change in a predictor variable, after taking into account the other predictor variables in the model. Odds ratios that are greater than one indicate that there is a greater likelihood of falling into the baseline outcome category (i.e., precontemplation in our examples) given an increase of one point in the specific predictor variable associated with the odds ratio. Odds ratios that are less than one indicate that there is less likelihood of falling into the baseline outcome category when the value for a specific predictor variable is increased by one point. In contrast to both MR and DFA, then, larger (odds ratio) values are associated with predictors that are more strongly linked with the lower stages (e.g., precontemplatión) than predictors with smaller values that are associated with higher level stages (e.g., maintenance). To make interpretation similar across the different methods, we reverse the ordering of the stage categories to make the baseline or reference category be the highest stage of maintenance in our example near the end of this chapter (see section on What Is an Example of Applying LR to a Research Question?).

HOW DO CENTRAL THEMES OF VARIANCE, COVARIANCE, AND LINEAR COMBINATIONS APPLY TO LR?

Although LR still focuses to some degree on a linear combination similar to MR (e.g., see equations 4.1 and 4.2 in the MR Chapter 4), the function that is modeled with LR is nonlinear (i.e., see equations 9.1 and 9.3, above). LR is also concerned with shared variance between the IVs and the DV, though a traditional R^2 value is not always standard output with LR, whereas it is regularly given for MR and even analysis of variance (ANOVA). Similarly, we are concerned with covariances among IVs with LR, especially when considering possible collinearity. However, we do not conventionally focus on or provide correlations (i.e., standardized covariances) among variables in LR output.

   In contrast to multivariate analysis of variance (MANOVA) or DFA, LR, like MR and analysis of covariance (ANCOVA), does not involve eigenvalues or eigenvector weights. Still, the central themes of variance, covariance and linear combinations play a part in LR as we will see below with macro- and micro-level assessment.

WHAT ARE THE MAIN THEMES NEEDED TO INTERPRET LR RESULTS AT A MACRO-LEVEL?

At a macro-level, LR is no different than other methods we have considered previously (e.g., MR, ANCOVA, MANOVA, and DFA). We would always want to begin with examining a macro-level significance test and effect size. As a preliminary step, however, LR should begin with a test of a proportional odds assumption whenever the DV has more than two categories. This assumption assesses whether the odds ratios, the weights examined at the micro-level for LR (see section on What Are the Main Themes Needed to Interpret LR Results at a Micro-Level?), are proportional over different pairs of categories. Loosely similar to the homogeneity of regression assumption in ANCOVA, we would like the odds ratio weights to be similar regardless of the different pairs of categories. When this assumption does not hold, as we will see shortly in our example, we know that the logistic regression weights differ depending on the category groupings of the outcome. To explore this further, it is a good idea to conduct follow-up LR analyses with pairwise categories of the outcome variable. We see an application of this in the example presented later in section What Is an Example of Applying LR to a Research Question?

Significance test

For LR, we calculate the log-likelihood (LL) by:

$$LL = \text{sum of } [Y_i \times LN(X_i') + (1 - Y_i) \times LN(1 - X_i')], \qquad (9.4)$$

where $i = 1$ to N, and Y_i is the actual outcome score (i.e., 1 or 0) that is multiplied by the natural log of X_i' as defined in equation 9.3, which is then added to $1 - Y_i$ times the natural log of 1 minus a predicted X_i' score. The LL is usually calculated for a specific model, M, with a set of "p" predictors and an intercept, and is compared with the LL for a model (I) that includes only an intercept parameter (I) and no predictors. A chi-square significance test can then be calculated as:

$$\chi^2 = 2\,[LL\ (M) - LL\ (I)] \qquad (9.5)$$

If the chi-square for this difference in log-likelihoods is significant, we can conclude that the model with the set of p predictors is significantly better than the model that includes just an intercept constant.

Effect size

For LR, we do not usually get a traditional R^2 value accompanying a macro-level significance test. Several indices (e.g., Somer's D, gamma, tau-a, and c; and McFadden's ρ^2) are provided with some computer packages (e.g., SAS, and SPSS, respectively). The values differ in how they deal with pairs of outcome categories, and the range of values for the index, with McFadden's ρ^2 being the most conservative, and c usually having the largest values (i.e., a range of 0.5 to 1.0). To calculate an effect size (ES) that can be interpreted as the proportion of shared variance between a set of predictors and a categorical outcome, it may be best to average several indices. This maintains the spirit of multiplicity, recognizing that we often need multiple measures or methods to estimate a single underlying concept (e.g., shared variance). This average shared variance index can be evaluated with Cohen's (1992) guidelines for a multivariate ES (i.e., 0.02, 0.13, and 0.26 for small, medium, and large effect sizes, respectively). A formula for one of the R^2-like indices is given below:

$$\text{McFadden's } \rho^2 = 1 - [LL\ (M)/LL\ (I)], \qquad (9.6)$$

where LL(M) is the log-likelihood for a specific model with p predictors, and LL (I) is the log-likelihood for a model that only includes an intercept parameter or constant.

When we get a significant χ^2 test and a reasonable ES, it is worthwhile to examine specific micro-level findings to assess which variables are significant in predicting membership in the outcome.

WHAT ARE THE MAIN THEMES NEEDED
TO INTERPRET LR RESULTS
AT A MICRO-LEVEL?

Predictor variables can be evaluated in at least two ways with LR:

a. **Logistic regression weights and significance tests.** The initial weights that come out of an LR analysis can be evaluated for significance much like what is done in MR. The significance test for these weights is a Wald test that is interpreted as a z- or t-test and is simply the ratio of the LR coefficient divided by its standard error. Some computer programs use a χ^2 test to assess the significance of weights.

b. **Odds ratios.** It is useful to examine the odds of falling into an outcome category given a one-unit change in a specific predictor. These odds ratios are calculated for each predictor and are helpful when interpreting which IVs provide relevant information in predicting membership in the outcome variable. Larger values for an odds ratio associated with an IV indicate that participants with high scores on that IV have greater odds of falling into the baseline reference category. The reference category is usually the highest category (i.e., the one coded with a 1 versus a 0 in a dichotomous outcome). Because some computer routines (e.g., SAS, 1999) use the smallest category as a reference, it is useful to flip the valence to a descending order to be consistent with other programs and interpretation (e.g., focus on the likelihood of falling into the fifth stage of condom use, maintenance, instead of the first stage, precontemplation). To aid in interpretation, we use this reversed, descending order of the outcome categories in the example presented later.

WHAT ARE SOME OTHER
CONSIDERATIONS OR NEXT
STEPS AFTER APPLYING LR?

After conducting an LR analysis, caution should be applied, especially if the exploratory model-building format was adopted. Results are more reliable when they have been confirmed on an independent sample from which a model was initially explored. As always, without random assignment to groups, manipulation of variables, and longitudinal designs, none of which is common with LR, it is difficult to impossible to ascribe causality.

With LR, as with many other methods, we also want to evaluate the reliability of our measures and whether we had included adequate covariates or confounding variables. The latter variables would help in ruling out alternative explanations for the findings. Finally, the nature of the sample should be evaluated as to its size, its relevance to the phenomenon under study, and its ability to provide relatively generalizable results.

WHAT IS AN EXAMPLE OF APPLYING LR TO A RESEARCH QUESTION?

Output is provided below for LR using the same variables and time points as in the DFA stand-alone example (and the same variables, though different time point for the IVs in the standard MR example). As before, the four predictor IVs are psychosexual functioning, pros of condom use, cons of condom use, and condom self-efficacy. The outcome is stage of condom use. To include a longitudinal aspect, the IVs are measured at the first time point (i.e., indicated by the letter A at the end of each variable name), and the outcome is measured 6 months later (i.e., indicated by the letter B at the end of the outcome name, STAGEB). There is no need to repeat the preliminary descriptives and correlations that were presented earlier (see stand-alone example in the DFA chapter). As with previous examples, the LR analysis draws on both the transtheoretical model (e.g., Prochaska et al., 1994) and the multifaceted model of HIV risk (Harlow et al., 1993).

Several LR analyses were conducted where the nature of the categorical DV changed for each analysis. In the first analysis, the outcome has five levels (i.e., the five stages of condom use). For the last four analyses, four dichotomous outcome variables are created to compare stages 2 to 5, respectively, with the first stage, precontemplation (coded 0 in each dichotomy). Because there are varying numbers of participants in each of the five stages, the sample sizes vary for the four analyses with a dichotomous outcome (see calculations, below). These four LRs with dichotomous outcomes can be viewed as follow-up analyses to the initial LR to determine with which stage levels the predictors were most significantly related. Given the multiple analyses, it is probably wise to use a more conservative alpha level such as 0.01 for the four follow-up analyses, with the conventional 0.05 alpha level for the initial analysis.

a. The first LR analysis uses the same five-level (stage of condom use at time B: STAGEB) DV as was used in MR and in DFA.
b. The second LR analysis uses a dichotomous STAGE2B DV, with precontemplators coded 0 and individuals in the second stage, contemplators, coded 1.
c. The third analysis uses a dichotomous STAGE3B DV, with precontemplation coded as 0 and individuals in the third stage, preparation, coded as 1.
d. The fourth LR analysis again codes a dichotomous STAGE4B DV as 0 for precontemplation, but a 1 is now given for those in the fourth action stage of condom use.

TABLE 9.1
Frequencies for STAGEB for LR Example

The LOGISTIC Procedure Response Profile

Ordered Value	Total STAGEB	Frequency
1 = Maintenance	5	87
2 = Action	4	22
3 = Preparation	3	79
4 = Contemplation	2	185
5 = Precontemplation	1	154

e. Finally, the last LR analysis uses a dichotomous STAGE5B DV with those in the fifth stage, maintenance, coded as 1, with the same baseline of pre-contemplators coded as 0.

LR Results for 5-Stage DV

The first part of the output for the LR example provides the frequencies for the five response categories for the outcome, STAGEB. As we have noticed from previous chapters, there are highly discrepant sample sizes per group, which is not optimal. Notice also that we reordered the Stages in "descending" order so that our odds ratios can be interpreted with respect to the highest stage (i.e., Stage 5 = maintenance for the first analysis).

From the list of frequencies for each stage (see Table 9.1), we can ascertain the sample sizes for each LR analysis. For the first LR analysis with the five-category outcome, $N = 527$ because data from all participants are used. For the second LR comparing contemplators and precontemplators, we have $N = 185 + 154 = 339$. For the third LR, comparing those in preparation with precontemplators, $N = 79 + 154 = 233$. For the fourth LR (including those in Stage 4, action, and Stage 1, precontemplation) we have $N = 154 + 22 = 176$; for the fifth LR (comparing those in Stage 5, maintenance, and Stage 1, precontemplation) our sample size is $N = 87 + 154 = 241$.

Table 9.2 provides results for a test of an initial assumption needed when conducting LR on an outcome with more than two categories. Findings for the proportional odds assumption (labeled a "score test" in SAS, 1999) indicate that the odds ratios between similar stage categories are significantly different. This is not ideal and suggests that the likelihood of falling in one of the stage categories, given the set of four predictors, is not proportional. This could be due to the disproportionate sample sizes for the stage categories and/or to the fact that the four IVs may not be as effective in predicting membership into some of the stages. We saw this with DFA classification results, where membership in the extreme

TABLE 9.2

Initial Test of Odds Assumption for Five-Stage DV

Score Test for the Proportional Odds Assumption

Chi-Square	DF	Pr > ChiSq
26.6002	12	0.0088

stages (i.e., precontemplation and maintenance) was more easily predicted than for, say, the second (i.e., contemplation) stage of condom use. Although the lack of proportionality is not optimal, we will proceed cautiously with interpreting the output from this LR analysis.

In Table 9.3, notice that the likelihood ratio is significant $[\chi^2(4) = 183.2448, p < 0.0001]$, indicating that the model with both the intercept and four predictors (i.e., Model M) is better than the model with the intercept only (i.e., Model I).

Table 9.4 presents four macro-level indices that can be interpreted as a correlation between the set of IVs and the DV. A macro-level effect size can be calculated by squaring any of the indices in the far right column of Table 9.4. Because these produce discrepant values (i.e., 0.24, 0.25, 0.13, and 0.56, respectively for squared values of Somer's D, gamma, tau-a, and c), it is also useful to calculate McFadden's ρ^2 (see equation 9.4):

$$\text{McFadden's } \rho^2 = 1 - [\text{LL (M)/LL (I)}] = 1 - (1336.025/1519.270)$$

$$= 1 - 0.879386 = 0.12$$

Using Cohen's (1992) guidelines, this represents approximately a medium multivariate effect size (similar to the value obtained by squaring tau-a, above). This

TABLE 9.3

Macro-Level LR Results for Five-Stage DV

	Model Fit Statistics	
Criterion	*Intercept Only* *[Model I]*	*Intercept and IVs* *[Model M]*
AIC	1527.270	1352.025
SC	1544.338	1386.163
−2 Log L	1519.270	1336.025

Testing Global Null Hypothesis: BETA = 0

Test	Chi-Square	DF	Pr > Chi-Sq.
Likelihood Ratio	183.2448	4	<0.0001
Score	154.4480	4	<0.0001
Wald	155.4034	4	<0.0001

TABLE 9.4
Macro-Level Indices for LR with Five-Stage DV

Association of Predicted Probabilities and Observed Responses with 4 LR Indices

Percent Concordant	74.4	Somers' D	0.493
Percent Discordant	25.1	Gamma	0.495
Percent Tied	0.5	Tau-a	0.365
Pairs	102747	c	0.746

---

is substantially smaller than the multivariate effect size found with a DFA (i.e., $\eta^2 = 1 - \Lambda = 0.32$) or MR (i.e., $R^2 = 0.29$) of these same data (see DFA and MR chapters). This is probably because LR is not as powerful as either DFA or MR. Given the range of values for the macro-level effect sizes from Somer's D, gamma, tau-a, c, and McFadden's ρ^2, as suggested earlier it might be useful to average these to arrive at a more balanced assessment of the proportion of shared variance between the linear combination of predictors and the outcome. The average of these five indices provides a moderately large ES, a value that is more in line with that found from DFA and MR:

$$(0.24 + 0.25 + 0.13 + 0.56 + 0.12)/5 = 0.25.$$

Thus, we could conclude that the four predictors for this LR analysis explain approximately 25% of the variance in stage of condom use.

An inspection of the significance tests (i.e., chi-square) and probabilities for the LR parameter estimates (see Table 9.5) reveals that all four of the predictors are significantly predicting membership in the outcome variable, StageB (at the conservative alpha level of .01 or better). Thus, it is helpful to examine the odds ratios for each predictor.

The pattern of odds ratios in Table 9.6 indicates that individuals who score high in psychosexual functioning are only half as likely to fall in the maintenance stage

TABLE 9.5
Micro-Level LR Results for Five-Stage DV

		Analysis of Maximum Likelihood Estimates			
Parameter	*DF*	*Estimate*	*Standard Error*	*Chi-Square*	*Pr > Chi-Sq.*
Intercept	1	−2.3209	0.6906	11.2942	0.0008
Intercept2	1	−1.9812	0.6892	8.2629	0.0040
Intercept3	1	−1.0361	0.6869	2.2753	0.1315
Intercept4	1	0.8601	0.6838	1.5818	0.2085
PSYSXA	1	−0.6721	0.1139	34.8353	<0.0001
PROSA	1	0.3474	0.0939	13.6820	0.0002
CONSA	1	−0.2842	0.1038	7.5020	0.0062
CONSEFFA	1	0.6876	0.0781	77.4682	<0.0001

TABLE 9.6
Micro-Level Odds Ratio Estimates for LR with Five-Stage DV

		Odds Ratio Estimates	
			95% Wald
Effect	*Point Estimate*		*Confidence Limits*
PSYSXA	0.511	0.408	0.638
PROSA	1.415	1.177	1.701
CONSA	0.753	0.614	0.922
CONSEFFA	1.989	1.707	2.318

of condom use (than in earlier stages). Similarly, but to a slightly larger degree, individuals who score high on the cons of condom use are about three-quarters as likely to be staged in maintenance (and thus are more likely to be classified into an earlier stage). Conversely, individuals who score high in condom self-efficacy are almost twice as likely to be in the maintenance stage of condom use, and those scoring high on the pros of condom use are 1.4 times more likely to fall in the maintenance category as in one of the earlier stages. Although the nature of these values is not the same as that of the loadings in DFA or the standardized regression coefficients in MR, the interpretation of the findings is similar. Condom self-efficacy appears to be the most salient predictor of who will have a high stage (i.e., maintenance) of condom use. Figure 9.1 depicts the LR prediction model for this five-stage DV with odds ratios provided for each IV.

We now turn to the first follow-up LR analysis that explores whether the same four IVs (psychosexual functioning, pros, cons, and condom self-efficacy) can predict a dichotomous outcome comparing contemplators (score = 1) to

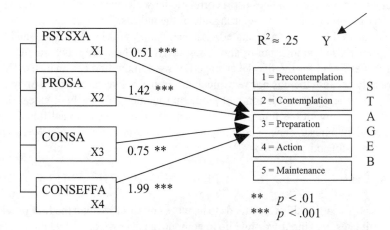

FIG. 9.1.   LR predicting five-stage DV with odds ratios provided.

TABLE 9.7
Frequencies for STAGE2B for LR Example (DV: 1 = Contemplation
vs. 0 = Precontemplation)

		The LOGISTIC Procedure Response Profile
Variable Name	Code for STAGE2B	Total Frequency
Contemplation	1	185
Precontemplation	0	154

precontemplators (i.e., score = 0). Given the initial significance of the proportional odds (i.e., score) test earlier, it is likely that LR results will vary for the four follow-up analyses, depending on the stages compared in the dichotomous outcomes.

LR Results for Dichotomous STAGE2B DV (Stage 2 Versus 1)

Table 9.7 gives the frequencies for individuals in Stages 2 and 1 of the dichotomous DV, STAGE2B analyzed here. Note that the frequencies are approximately equal across the two stage categories, but only a total of 339 participants (i.e., those in Stages 2 and 1) were analyzed.

Table 9.8 provides the macro-level test results for this follow-up LR with STAGE2B as a dichotomous DV. As with the five-level DV, we conclude that the model (M) with predictors and intercept provides a better fit than the model (I) with only the intercept.

Table 9.9 presents four macro-level indices for the model with STAGE2B. Remembering that these indices use a correlational scale, we can obtain estimates of a macro-level effect size by squaring any of the indices. These calculations would yield squared (proportion of shared variance) values of 0.11, 0.11, 0.03, and 0.44 for Somer's D, gamma, tau-a, and c, respectively. These are much smaller than the values found for the five-level stage DV used in the first LR analysis. This is probably because there is not very much difference between the stages of precontemplation and contemplation and predicting membership in these categories is not as precise with the four predictors analyzed (i.e., psychosexual functioning, pros of condom use, cons of condom use, and condom self-efficacy). We can also calculate McFadden's ρ^2 as:

$$\text{McFadden's } \rho^2 = 1 - [\text{LL (M)}/\text{LL (C)}] = 1 - 435.751/467.115 = 0.07$$

As noted earlier, this value tends to be more conservative than the four previous ES estimates, making it worthwhile to compute an average of all five indices (i.e., Somer's D, gamma, tau-a, c, and McFadden's ρ^2) to get a more robust estimate

TABLE 9.8
Macro-Level LR Results for STAGE2B Example
(DV: 1 = Contemplation vs. 0 = Precontemplation)

	Model Fit Statistics	
Criterion	*Intercept Only* [Model I]	*Intercept and IVs* [Model M]
AIC	469.115	445.751
SC	472.941	464.881
−2 Log L	467.115	435.751

Testing Global Null Hypothesis: BETA = 0

Test	*Chi-Square*	*DF*	*Pr > Chi-Sq.*
Likelihood Ratio	31.3638	4	<0.0001
Score	30.1529	4	<0.0001
Wald	27.9613	4	<0.0001

(i.e., the average of 0.11, 0.11, 0.03, 0.44, and 0.07 = 0.15). This represents a medium multivariate effect size by Cohen's (1992) standards and indicates that it would be worthwhile to further explore the nature of prediction by examining the micro-level weights (both unstandardized and odds ratios).

Table 9.10 gives the micro-level results for the parameter estimates for predicting STAGE2B. Note that the predictor, CONSA, is not significant, and the predictor, PROSA, is not significant at the conservative 0.01 level set for follow-up analyses. The other two predictors, psychosexual functioning and condom self-efficacy are significant. Thus, we would interpret only the odds ratio estimates for these latter two predictors (see Figure 9.2). The findings with this dichotomous DV contrasting contemplators with precontemplators are similar in nature, if not the exact magnitude, as those from the five-level stage DV. In the current analysis, an individual with high condom self-efficacy is 1.36 times more likely to fall in a higher stage of condom use. Conversely, those with a high psychosexual functioning score are just a little more than half as likely to fall into a higher stage of

TABLE 9.9
Macro-Level LR Indices for STAGE2B Example
(DV: 1 = Contemplation vs. 0 = Precontemplation)

Association of Predicted Probabilities and Observed Responses with 4 LR Indices

Percent Concordant	66.4	Somers' D	0.331
Percent Discordant	33.3	Gamma	0.332
Percent Tied	0.3	Tau-a	0.165
Pairs	28490	c	0.666

TABLE 9.10
Micro-Level LR Results for STAGE2B Example (DV: 1 = Contemplation vs.
0 = Precontemplation)

Parameter	DF	Estimate	Standard Error	Chi-Square	Pr >Chi-Sq.
		Analysis of Maximum Likelihood Estimates			
Intercept	1	0.6467	0.9488	0.4646	0.4955
PSYSXA	1	−0.5193	0.1685	9.4933	0.0021
PROSA	1	0.2923	0.1185	6.0851	0.0136
CONSA	1	−0.1289	0.1462	0.7783	0.3777
CONSEFFA	1	0.3058	0.1027	8.8673	0.0029

condom use. It is also interesting to note that the values for the two nonsignificant odds ratios (i.e., for PROSA and CONSA) are similar across the LR analyses
conducted with the five-level and two-level DVs, respectively. Because PROSA
and CONSA were significant predictors in the initial analysis that included the
full sample of individuals at all five stages, we could surmise that there was most
likely not enough power to find significance for these two predictors in the current
analysis that included less than two-thirds of the original sample. This lack of
power is apt to be even more of a concern for subsequent analyses that include
even smaller proportions of the full sample. Of course, we cannot rule out the possibility that PROSA and CONSA simply do not do well in differentiating between
precontemplators and contemplators of condom use. Thus, although macro- and
micro-level decisions are somewhat similar across the two ways of scoring the
categorical DV, there is much less shared variance and fewer significant predictors

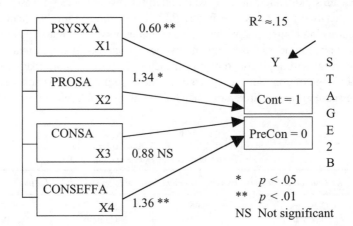

FIG. 9.2. LR predicting contemplation versus precontemplation
with odds ratios provided.

TABLE 9.11

Frequencies for STAGE3B for LR Example (DV: 1 = Preparation vs. 0 = Precontemplation)

	Response Profile	
Variable Name	Code for STAGE3B	Total Frequency
Preparation	1	79
Precontemplation	0	154

with this follow-up comparing those who are thinking about using condoms versus those who are not even considering condoms.

We now explore the nature of prediction when using the same four IVs (psychosocial functioning, pros, cons, and condom self-efficacy) to predict membership in a dichotomous DV where individuals in Stage 3 (preparation) are coded "1" and individuals in Stage 1 (precontemplation) are coded "0".

LR Results for Dichotomous STAGE3B DV (Stage 3 Versus 1)

Table 9.11 presents the frequencies for the two categories for the dichotomous DV, STAGE3B. Note that there are only a total of 233 participants analyzed, with the preparation stage being almost half the size of the precontemplation stage. Thus, this follow-up LR may not yield very robust results given the uneven sample sizes.

Table 9.12 presents the macro-level results for the LR model with STAGE3B as the dichotomous DV. Because the likelihood ratio chi-square statistic is significant,

TABLE 9.12

Macro-Level LR Results for STAGE3B Example (DV: 1 = Preparation vs. 0 = Precontemplation)

	Model Fit Statistics		
Criterion	Intercept Only [Model I]		Intercept and IVs [Model M]
AIC	300.430		247.973
SC	303.881		265.228
−2 Log L	298.430		237.973
	Testing Global Null Hypothesis: BETA = 0		
Test	Chi-Square	DF	Pr > Chi-Sq.
Likelihood Ratio	60.4571	4	<0.0001
Score	53.3190	4	<0.0001
Wald	41.6045	4	<0.0001

TABLE 9.13

Macro-Level LR Indices for STAGE3B Example (DV: 1 = Preparation vs.
0 = Precontemplation)

Association of Predicted Probabilities and Observed Responses with 4 LR Indices

Percent Concordant	79.0	Somers' D	0.582
Percent Discordant	20.8	Gamma	0.584
Percent Tied	0.2	Tau-a	0.262
Pairs	12166	c	0.791

we can conclude that a model (M) with the four predictors and the intercept is better than a model (I) with only the intercept for this analysis comparing those in the preparation stage of condom use with those in the precontemplation stage. From the values in this table, we can also calculate McFadden's $\rho^2 = 1 - 237.973/298.430 = 0.20$, which represents a medium-large multivariate ES.

Table 9.13 gives the values for the other four macro-level indices for this LR. As in previous LR analyses, we can calculate an estimate of the macro-level ES by squaring the values for Somer's D, gamma, tau-a, and c and averaging them with the value for McFadden's ρ^2. This average ES can be calculated as:

$$(0.58^2 + 0.58^2 + 0.26^2 + 0.79^2 + 0.20)/5 = 1.5645/5 = 0.31.$$

This represents a large ES for predicting membership in preparation versus precontemplation, in contrast to the previous follow-up LR analysis (i.e., ES = 0.15 when contrasting contemplators and precontemplators). It is also slightly larger than what was found when analyzing all five stages with the full sample (i.e., ES = 0.25). Thus, it appears that the four IVs do a better job at predicting membership in either preparation or precontemplation than when predicting membership in the five-level stage DV or the contemplation versus precontemplation DV. It would now be helpful to assess which predictors were most clearly related to predicting membership into either preparation or precontemplation.

Figure 9.3 summarizes the micro-level results for this LR analysis with STAGE3B by providing the odds ratios for the four predictors and their corresponding levels of significance. A slightly different pattern emerges than what we saw from the earlier LR analyses. Here, the individuals who are high in perceiving the pros of condom use and in condom self-efficacy are about one and three-quarters as likely to be staged in preparation versus precontemplation. Thus, pros takes a much more predominant role in this middle Stage 3 category. As with earlier analyses, individuals high in psychosexual functioning are not very likely to be in a high stage of condom use, even though the value for the odds ratio is even smaller (i.e., 0.39) than what was found previously (i.e., 0.60 and 0.51 for the

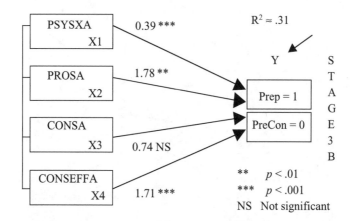

FIG. 9.3. LR predicting preparation versus precontemplation with odds ratios provided.

five-level DV and the dichotomy of contemplation and precontemplation stages). Finally, cons is not a significant predictor, as was the case in the previous follow-up LR analysis.

Next, we present the highlights for the LR analysis contrasting those in action with those in precontemplation for condom use.

LR Results for Dichotomous STAGE4B DV (Stage 4 Versus 1)

In this follow-up LR analysis, the same four predictors (i.e., psychosexual functioning, pros of condom use, cons of condom use, and condom self-efficacy) are used to predict the likelihood of falling in either the fourth stage, action, versus the first stage of precontemplation. The sample sizes are highly discrepant for this analysis with only 22 participants in action contrasted with the group of precontemplators that is a full 7 times the size (i.e., $n1 = 154$). Results should be viewed cautiously for at least two reasons: (1) the total sample size is 176, which is not quite 50 times the number of IVs (i.e., $N \geq 200$ is preferred with this LR); and (2) the stark difference in sample sizes may well yield results that are neither stable nor robust. Still, it is worth exploring this follow-up LR analysis to see whether any insight can be gained as to how to differentiate those in action versus those in precontemplation for condom use in a sample of at-risk women.

For convenience, tabular results are avoided with the main highlights presented in the text and in a figure. As with previous analyses, the likelihood chi-square for the model (M) that included predictors and an intercept was significantly better than the model (I) with only the intercept (i.e, likelihood $\chi^2(4) = 20.8150$,

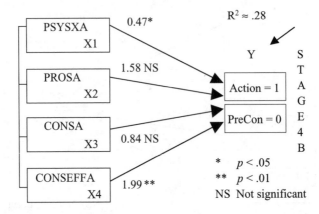

FIG. 9.4. LR predicting action versus precontemplation with odds ratios provided.

$p = 0.0003$). The estimates of shared variance between the four predictors and the outcome dichotomy (i.e., action versus precontemplation) produced a large ES when averaging values from (Somer's $D)^2$, (gamma)^2, (tau-$a)^2$, $(c)^2$, and McFadden's ρ^2 =, respectively:

$$(0.562^2 + 0.565^2 + 0.124^2 + 0.781^2 + 0.16)/5 = 1.4215/5 \approx 0.28.$$

The substantial proportion of shared variance merits an examination of the micro-level findings (i.e., odds ratios and significance levels) presented in Figure 9.4. Notice that only one of the predictors, condom self-efficacy, meets the stringent 0.01 level of significance. This is most likely due to the incredibly small sample size for the action stage (i.e., $n4 = 22$) providing too little power to detect significance. This speculation bears true, particularly for the IV pros of condom use, which has a larger odds ratio in this analysis (i.e., 1.58) than in the initial LR on the full sample size when the odds ratio was 1.42, which was significant at $p < 0.001$ previously. Still, the best that we can conclude from the current LR analysis is that individuals who are high in condom self-efficacy are just about two times as likely to be in the action stage of condom use, as those in precontemplation.

We now turn to the final LR, presenting the main findings when comparing those in Stage 5, maintenance ($n5 = 87$), with those in Stage 1, precontemplation ($n1 = 154$). As with all the earlier analyses, the same four predictors are used (i.e., psychosexual functioning, pros of condom use, cons of condom use, and condom self-efficacy). Similarly, we adhere to an alpha level of 0.05 for the macro-level results and an alpha level of 0.01 for micro-level findings.

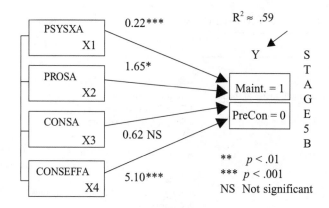

FIG. 9.5. LR predicting maintenance versus precontemplation with odds ratios provided.

LR Results for Dichotomous STAGE5B DV (Stage 5 Versus 1)

As with the previous LR follow-up analysis, tabled results are avoided in favor of a brief summary in the text and in a figure. Macro-level findings reveal, similar to before, that the likelihood chi-square for the full model (M: with predictors and intercept) fits significantly better than a model (I) that includes only the intercept [i.e., likelihood χ^2 (4) = 153.7367, p < 0.0001]. A macro-level ES can be calculated, as before, by squaring the four values provided in the SAS (1999) output (i.e., Somer's D, gamma, tau-a, and c) and averaging them with the value for McFadden's ρ^2 (i.e., $1 - 161.486/315.223 = 0.49$):

$$ES = (0.847^2 + 0.848^2 + 0.392^2 + 0.924^2 + 0.49)/5 \approx 0.59.$$

This represents a very large effect size, with more than half of the variance in STAGE5B membership (i.e., maintenance versus precontemplation) shared with the set of four predictors. It is certainly appropriate to examine micro-level findings.

Figure 9.5 shows only two significant predictors at the 0.01 level. The odds ratio for condom self-efficacy indicates that an individual who scores high on this predictor is more than five times as likely to be in the maintenance stage of condom use as in the precontemplation stage. Similar to what was found in previous analyses, those who score high in psychosexual functioning are highly unlikely to be staged in maintenance.

Extrapolating from all five of the LR analyses, it appears that individuals who are high in condom self-efficacy are most likely to be in the maintenance stage

TABLE 9.14
Multiplicity, Background, Central, and Interpretation Themes Applied to LR

Themes	Logistic Regression
Multiplicity themes (Note: + means multiplicity of theme pertains)	*+Theory, hypotheses and empirical Research* *+Controls*: covariate(s) *+Time Points*: IVs and/or DV *+Samples*: Cross validate *+Measurements*: +IVs, 1 categorical DV, (+covariates)
Background themes	*Sample data*: random selection *Measures*: grouping DV, grouping or continuous IVs and covariate(s) *Assumptions*: linear model assumptions not needed for descriptive use Large samples needed for greater power with maximum likelihood Exclusive and exhaustive DV categories required *Methods*: inferential with assumptions met
Central themes	*Variance*: in DV *Covariance*: among DVs and covariate(s) *Ratio*: likelihood
Interpretation themes	*Macro*: log-likelihood significance, ES = average of (Somer's D)^2, gamma^2, (tau-a)^2, c^2, and McFadden's ρ^2 *Micro:* coefficients, Wald tests, odds ratios
(Questions to ask)	What is probability of DV given set of IVs and covariates? Are all variables reliable and needed? Low correlations among IVs (i.e., no collinearity)? Significant ρ^2 or shared variance between IVs and DV? Compare different models to predict DV? Which IVs significantly increase probability of DV? Generalizability of results?

of condom use. In contrast, individuals who are high in psychosexual functioning are much more likely to not even be considering condom use (i.e., be in Stage 1, precontemplation). This suggests that those with a more positive sense of their sexuality are less likely to think they need to use condoms, possibly because they believe they are in long-term relationships with monogamous and low-risk partners. Perceiving the advantages of using condoms (i.e., pros) is most important in differentiating those in preparation versus those in precontemplation, whereas perceiving the disadvantages of condom use (i.e., cons) does not appear as important as any of the other predictors in differentiating across the stages of condom use.

SUMMARY

A summary of the various themes for LR is presented in Table 9.14.

REFERENCES

Aldrich, J. H., & Nelson, F. D. (1984). *Linear probability, logit, and probit models.* Beverly Hills, CA: Sage.

Cohen, J. (1992). A power primer. *Psychological Bulletin, 112,* 155–159.

Harlow, L. L., Quina, K., Morokoff, P. J., Rose, J. S., & Grimley, D. (1993). HIV risk in women: A multifaceted model. *Journal of Applied Biobehavioral Research, 1,* 3–38.

Hosmer, D. W., & Lemeshow, S. (1989). *Applied logistic regression.* New York: Wiley.

Menard, S. (1995). *Applied logistic regression analysis* (Sage University Paper 106 in the Series: Quantitative Applications in the Social Sciences). Thousand Oaks, CA: Sage Publications.

Prochaska, J. O., Velicer, W. F., Rossi, J. S., Goldstein, M. G., Marcus, B. H., Rakowski, W., Fiore, C., Harlow, L. L., Redding, C. A., Rosenbloom, D., & Rossi, S. R. (1994). Stages of change and decisional balance for 12 problem behaviors. *Health Psychology, 13,* 39–46.

Rose, J. S., Chassin, L., Presson, C. C., & Sherman, S. J. (2000) Prospective predictors of smoking cessation: A logistic regression application. In J. S. Rose, L. Chassin, C. C. Presson, & S. J. Sherman (Eds.), *Multivariate applications in substance use research* (Chapter 10: pp. 289–317). Mahwah, NJ: Lawrence Erlbaum Associates.

SAS (1999). *Statistical Analysis Software, Release 8.1.* Cary, NC: SAS Institute Inc.

Tabachnick, B. G., & Fidell, L. S. (2001). *Using multivariate statistics* (4th ed.) (Chapter 12: pp. 517–581). Boston: Allyn and Bacon.

Wright, R. E. (1995). Logistic regression. In L. G. Grimm & P. R. Yarnold (Eds.), *Reading and understanding multivariate statistics* (pp. 217–244). Washington, DC: American Psychological Association.

V

Multivariate Correlation Methods with Continuous Variables

10

Canonical Correlation

Themes Applied to Canonical Correlation (CC)

Canonical correlation is a very general multivariate method that allows multiple independent and multiple dependent variables. In this sense, CC subsumes other methods discussed so far and at one time was considered the penultimate multivariate method. With the development of even more encompassing multivariate methods, such as structural equation modeling, CC has been superceded in its status. Still, CC is an excellent exploratory method when investigating whether two sets of variables are related. It is also a good procedure for highlighting many of the statistical features we see in most multivariate methods. If we understand CC, we are much closer to having an overarching understanding of all the multivariate methods discussed in this book. More description of CC is presented in a number of excellent references (e.g., Campbell & Taylor, 1996; Cohen, Cohen, West, & Aiken, 2003; Fan, 1997; Tabachnick & Fidell, 2001; Takane & Hwang, 2002; Thompson, 2000; Thorndike, 2000).

Next, we approach CC with the same set of 10 questions that address how the themes apply to this multivariate method.

WHAT IS CC AND HOW IS IT SIMILAR TO AND DIFFERENT FROM OTHER METHODS?

CC is an extension of bivariate correlation that allows two or more usually continuous independent variables (IVs) (i.e., referred to as variables on the left) and two or more (usually continuous) dependent variables (DVs) (i.e., referred to as variables on the right). The focus is on correlations and weights, as opposed to group means or classification. The main question is how are the best linear combinations of the IVs related to the best linear combinations of the DVs? In CC, there are several layers of analysis:

a. We would like to explore whether pairs of linear combinations (i.e., labeled as canonical variates in CC) are significantly related;
b. We are interested in how the variables on the left (i.e., IVs) relate to their respective canonical variates, and how the variables on the right (i.e., DVs) relate to their respective canonical variates;
c. We would like to see how the variables on each side relate to the canonical variates on the other side (i.e., this is somewhat misleadingly labeled "redundancy analysis").
d. We can conduct follow-up multiple regressions (MRs), one for each DV, using the full set of IVs from CC as the IVs in each MR. This will provide insight about specific relationships among the IVs and each DV. To protect Type I error rate, it may be preferred to use a conservative alpha level, 0.01, or a Bonferroni approach that divides the desired alpha level (e.g., 0.05) by the number of follow-up analyses (e.g., $p = 0.05/2 = 0.025$). Researchers instead may choose the more traditional alpha level, 0.05.

If the number of IVs is equal to p and the number of DVs is equal to q, then the number of canonical variates (i.e., linear combinations) on each side, and hence the number of cross-side correlations (i.e., canonical correlations), is equal to the minimum of p or q. For example, with three substance use variables on the left and two personality variables on the right, there would be two canonical variates to explain the variance on each side. The first step would be to explore whether canonical correlations between the two pairs of canonical variates were significantly different from zero. Next, the correlations (i.e., canonical loadings) between the three substance use variables and their two canonical variates would be examined, followed by a similar examination of the canonical loadings for the two personality variables on their two canonical variates. Finally, it would be helpful to see how the three substance use variables related to each of the two personality canonical variates and how the two personality variables related to each of the two substance use canonical variates. Figure 10.1 depicts the first two layers of analysis for this example. To examine redundancy, add lines from each X to each W, and from each Y to each V.

Follow-up MRs, one for each DV, are depicted in Figure 10.2 for this example. Notice that all three predictors (i.e., alcohol, marijuana, and hard drug use) are used to predict the first DV, distress, and then the second DV, self-esteem. These follow-up analyses could be conducted with a more conservative alpha level (e.g., $p < 0.01$) to help control the overall Type I error rate when conducting multiple analyses. However, researchers interested in increasing the power of their study

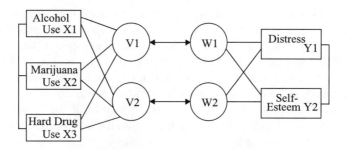

FIG. 10.1. CC with 3 Xs and 2 Ys, with each X linked to the 2 canonical variates, V1 and V2; and each Y linked to the 2 Ws. Connected lines for Xs and Ys represent possible correlation. Arrows between Vs and Ws indicate canonical correlations.

(and controlling Type II error) may choose the more conventional alpha level of $p < 0.05$ for both the CC and follow-up MRs.

CC is similar to MR in that multiple IVs are allowed. CC differs from MR in that MR allows only a single DV, whereas CC allows two or more DVs. CC is similar to discriminant function analysis (DFA) and logistic regression (LR) in that multiple IVs are allowed with all three methods. CC is different from both DFA and LR in that the latter two methods usually have only a single categorical

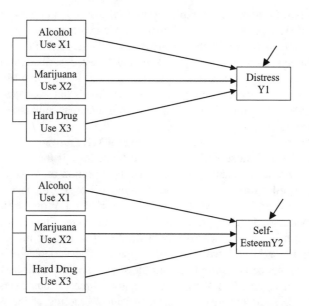

FIG. 10.2. Two follow-up MRs to further assess which Xs are linked with which Y. Connected lines for Xs represent possible correlation. The single arrow to Y represents prediction error.

outcome, whereas CC allows two or more usually continuous outcomes. CC is similar to analysis of covariance (ANCOVA) and multivariate analysis of variance (MANOVA) in requiring the general linear model assumptions (i.e., normality, linearity, and homoscedasticity) when making inferences to the population. CC differs from ANCOVA and MANOVA in that CC is a correlational method that does not have to include any categorical variables and is not focused on mean differences between groups. Finally, CC is similar to MR, DFA, and LR in its focus on weighted functions of the variables, where the most interpretable weights are correlational (ranging from -1.0 to $+1.0$).

As is probably obvious by this brief introduction, it is often difficult to interpret results with CC. The method is unstructured in nature, useful for exploring how two sets of variables are loosely related. Thus, CC is particularly helpful in newly emerging fields. It is sometimes preferable to use more focused methods (e.g., structural equation modeling), especially with more theoretically grounded areas, but that topic will be saved for another book.

WHEN IS CC USED AND WHAT RESEARCH QUESTIONS CAN IT ADDRESS?

CC has several main uses:

a. **CC can be used as an exploratory tool** to see if two sets of continuous variables are related (e.g., is alcohol, marijuana, and other drug use related to a set of psychosocial variables, such as distress and self-esteem)? If there is significant overall shared variance (i.e., by $1 - \Lambda \approx \eta^2$ and F-test, described further in section What Are the Main Themes Needed to Interpret CC Results at a Macro-Level?), several layers of analysis (see Figure 10.1) can show what variables are involved and the underlying dimensions or canonical variates that summarize the essence of these variables.

b. **CC can be used as a precursor to several MR analyses** whenever we have a number of DVs and several correlational predictors. If the macro-level CC is significant and has a meaningful effect size (see section on What Are the Main Themes Needed to Interpret CC Results at a Macro-Level?), then we can go on and conduct separate mid-level MR analyses, one for each DV on the right to assess which is better predicted by the set of IVs on the left (see Figure 10.2).

c. **CC can be used to assess how a single set of two or more variables is longitudinally related across two time points.** The variables collected at the initial time point serve as the IVs with the same variables collected at a second time point serving as the DVs. An examination of the various layers of analysis could provide some tentative evidence for causal ordering of the variables. An example of this is presented later in the chapter in section What Is an Example of Applying CC to a Research Question?

WHAT ARE THE MAIN MULTIPLICITY
THEMES FOR CC?

CC makes use of a number of multiplicity themes. Similar to the other methods we have examined, it is helpful to examine multiple theories and previous empirical studies before embarking on even the most exploratory CC. A researcher also would have to consider multiple IV constructs and multiple DV constructs, with reliable measures for each. The usual cautions about minimizing collinearity within sides (i.e., within IVs and within DVs) are even more important for CC given the multitude of variables involved. If the variables are too highly correlated within sides, the results could become unstable. It is also apparent that because there are several IVs and several DVs in a CC, a fairly large sample size is usually needed. A possible guideline is to double the amount of participants needed for a MR on only one set of the variables. As with any study, longitudinal data would extend the rigor of the conclusions, possibly allowing a researcher to begin disentangling the causal ordering of the variables. Of course, without an experimental design, it is difficult to have definitive causal evidence.

WHAT ARE THE MAIN BACKGROUND
THEMES APPLIED TO CC?

CC has background themes similar to, but more extensive than, MR. We would likely need a fairly large ($N \times$ p) data matrix with multiple (usually continuous) IVs and multiple (usually continuous) DVs. If possible, conduct a power analysis (see Cohen, 1988) to assess the number of participants that would be needed to detect the expected effects. As with all the methods examined so far, we should also calculate preliminary descriptive statistics and correlations among the variables. This should also include an assessment of the reliability of all variables. Finally, when wanting to make inferences beyond the sample used, it would be important to verify whether assumptions of normality, homoscedasticity, and linearity are met with the data.

WHAT IS THE STATISTICAL MODEL THAT
IS TESTED WITH CC?

For CC, we are interested in the matrices of correlation among the X (IV) and Y (DV) variables. The model can be written as follows:

$$\mathbf{Rcc} = \mathbf{Ryy}^{-1}\mathbf{Ryx}\ \mathbf{Rxx}^{-1}\mathbf{Rxy} \qquad (10.1)$$

The four submatrices needed for this analysis (i.e., $\mathbf{Ryy^{-1}}$, $\mathbf{Ryx}$, $\mathbf{Rxx^{-1}}$, and $\mathbf{Rxy}$) derive from partitioning the original larger matrix of correlations among the DVs and IVs into four sections. The first includes the inverse of the q by q matrix of correlations among the DVs. Second, we examine the correlations among the q DVs and the p IVs. Third, we take the inverse of the matrix of correlations among the p IVs. Finally, we multiply the three previous matrices by the p by q matrix of correlations among the IVs and DVs.

The nature of this model is further explained, below, when discussing ratios of (co-)variances.

HOW DO CENTRAL THEMES OF VARIANCE, COVARIANCE, AND LINEAR COMBINATIONS APPLY TO CC?

The central themes of variance, covariance, and linear combinations apply to CC in surprisingly comparable ways as for other methods with which we have some familiarity. An examination of equation 10.1 should reveal some similarity with the ratios examined for a simple bivariate correlation or even the F-test in analysis of variance (ANOVA). That is, we are focusing on the nature of the (standard-ized) covariance *between* two (sets of) variables divided by the (standardized) (co-)variation *within* a variable (set). That is, equation 10.1 is analogous to what we see in many statistical ratios:

$$(\text{Co})\textbf{variance between (groups or variables)}/ \qquad \qquad \\ (\text{the product of the}) \textbf{ variance within (groups or variables)} \qquad (10.2)$$

Thus, this is not too different from the formula for a correlation that examines the ratio of covariance of X and Y over the square root of the product of the variance of X and the variance of Y:

$$r = \text{covariance } (X \text{ and } Y)/\sqrt{[Variance(X)] \times [\text{variance}(Y)]} \qquad (10.3)$$

Similarly, it is not too far afield from the ratio of between-group variance over within-group variance that is examined with group difference methods such as ANOVA, ANCOVA, and MANOVA:

$$F = \text{variance between groups/variance within groups} \qquad (10.4)$$

The main difference between the ratio examined in CC and those with the other methods is that CC includes information on p multiple *independent* variables and q multiple *dependent* variables. As mentioned earlier, we can examine several linear combinations of the IVs and DVs, equal to whichever is smaller, p or q. This is not too different from what we found in MANOVA or DFA, with a couple of exceptions. First, we do not often have grouping variables in CC that necessitate forming dummy variables for $k - 1$ of the categories. Thus, we can form linear combinations for the smaller of the subset of vectors of data from the p IVs and from the q DVs. Second, because there are two full sets of variables, we want to have two sets of linear combinations, summarizing the IVs and the DVs, respectively. Thus, the total number of linear combinations in CC is equal to:

$$[2] \times [\text{minimum } (p, q)] \tag{10.5}$$

The total number of eigenvalues is equal to just the minimum of p or q because these represent the shared variance between pairs of linear combinations or canonical variates.

WHAT ARE THE MAIN THEMES NEEDED TO INTERPRET CC RESULTS AT A MACRO-LEVEL?

At a macro-level, CC (r_c) shows the degree of association between linear combinations of the variables on the left (IVs) and on the right (DVs). We have already seen that there is always more than one CC in a single analysis because several linear combinations may be formed on each side. That is, the number of CCs is equal to the minimum of p or q, the number of IVs and DVs, respectively. Because we always have at least two IVs and two DVs, there will always be at least two linear combinations per side and at least two CCs. Here is what is involved in macro- and mid-level steps:

a. **Is there a significant degree of relationship between sets of variables**? Check the overall F-test and summary criteria (i.e., Wilks's lambda, Pillai's trace, Hotelling-Lawley trace, and Roy's greatest characteristic root: GCR), as well as $1 - \Lambda \approx \eta^2$. If there is significance and a meaningful effect size (ES), move to next layer of analysis to see which pairs of canonical variates are significantly related. If this first overall relationship is significant, the first pair of canonical variates is also significantly related (i.e., this is the same test, similar to testing with DFA).

b. **Are the pairs of canonical variates significantly related and how much information in the variables is explained by each canonical variate**? Check (r_c^2) and associated F-tests. For each pair of canonical variates, there is an eigenvalue associated with it. One indication of the importance of each pair of variates is to calculate a proportion formed from an eigenvalue divided by the sum of all the eigenvalues. The sum of these proportions will necessarily add up to 1.0. Hence, they cannot be interpreted as proportion of variance terms but rather the proportion of available canonical variance attributable to that specific pair of variates. Most often, the first proportion reveals that the bulk of the variable information is in the first pair of canonical variates so that the others may not be worth examining. If a pair of canonical variates are significantly related and explain a large proportion of the variance in the variables, move to the next layer to see which variables are substantially related to each canonical variate.

WHAT ARE THE MAIN THEMES NEEDED TO INTERPRET CC RESULTS AT A MICRO-LEVEL?

a. **Are the variables related to underlying canonical variates**? In CC, as with DFA, there are three kinds of weights that could be examined. The first kind is an unstandardized eigenvector weight that is used when comparing weights across different samples. The second is a standardized weight, somewhat analogous to a standardized beta weight in MR. It differs from the beta weight, however, in that it may possibly extend past the range of -1 to $+1$ due to having multiple, and possibly an unequal number of, variables on each side. Thus, just as with DFA, the most interpretable weight is the third form, which is a canonical loading. A structure coefficient (i.e., canonical loading) ranges from -1 to $+1$ and shows how correlated each variable is with the respective canonical variate. This is like a part-whole relationship. Just as with DFA, variables with loadings of $|0.30|$ or greater are interpreted as having a meaningful part on the whole dimension. Try to interpret the nature of each dimension by what loads highly on it. The higher the absolute value of the loading, the more a variable is involved in the essence of the linear combination or canonical variate. Also take note of the sign attached to the loading: a negative loading indicates that a high score on the variable relates to a low score on the variate.

b. **Are variables on one side related to variates on the other side**? After examining loadings of variables on their respective variates, check redundancy indices (RIs) for each canonical variate. RIs tell us how related the variables on one side are to a canonical variate from the other side. As with loadings and other interpretable weights and correlations, we would like RI values of $|0.30|$ or greater. Still, it is rare to have RI values that are as high as loadings because the former relates variables on one side with variates on the other, whereas the latter relates variables and variates on the same side.

c. **Which DVs are significantly predicted from the set of IVs**? A good follow-up procedure after finding significant and meaningful results in CC is to conduct q MRs, one for each DV. This allows an assessment of how much of the variance in each DV can be explained by the set of IVs. If protecting the Type I error rate is important, it may be preferred to use a protected alpha level (e.g., a Bonferroni approach of alpha divided by q or a strict 0.01 alpha level) both for the overall F-test of the R^2 as well as the individual weights. Alternatively, a researcher could opt to increase power and reduce Type II error rate by maintaining an alpha level of 0.05, even for follow-up MRs.

WHAT ARE SOME OTHER CONSIDERATIONS OR NEXT STEPS AFTER APPLYING CC?

After conducting a CC, it is important to consider whether the design allows inferences beyond the specific sample involved. Because CC analyses are often used in exploratory or descriptive studies, it is unlikely that many inferences can be made. Still, with careful consideration of possible confounds, attention to assumptions, and use of longitudinal data, it may be possible to make some tentative inferences.

If results from a CC analysis seem promising, it would be useful to plan more rigorous investigations. This could involve a structural equation model of the data that tests theoretically justified hypotheses about the nature of the relationships. For example, we could posit several latent variables (e.g., factors), each with several variables that are related. We would then make predictions, anchored in theory and empirical research, among the latent factors. We would not be limited to the restricted pattern and number of relationships that are allowed only in CC. We could also consider conducting one or more experimental designs on some or all of the variables to investigate the nature of causality. This would be especially fruitful with variables that loaded highly on their respective variates as well as loading highly on variates on the opposite side.

WHAT IS AN EXAMPLE OF APPLYING CC TO A RESEARCH QUESTION?

For CC, we focus on the same five variables (psychosexual functioning, pros, cons, condom self-efficacy, and stage of condom use) we examined in previous chapter examples. To include *two* sets of variables, and allow a possible test of the causal ordering of the variables, longitudinal data will be examined. Data for the five variables collected at the onset of the study (i.e., at $t1$) will constitute the IVs, whereas data from the five variables collected 6 months later (i.e., at $t2$) will make up the DVs.

We rely on the same theory as previously, drawing on the transtheoretical model (e.g., Prochaska et al., 1994) and multifaceted model of HIV risk (Harlow et al., 1993). To provide a more thorough exploration of the data, several layers of analysis will be conducted, with output provided for each: A, correlations among the p IVs and q DVs; B, a macro-level assessment of CC; C, midlevel assessment of the canonical correlations among the pairs of canonical variates; D, micro-level assessment of canonical loadings for both IVs and DVs; E, micro-level assessment of the (redundancy) relationships among variables on one side and canonical variates on the other side; and F, follow-up MRs, one for each DV, to attempt to examine the directional ordering of the variables.

Correlations Among the p IVs and q DVs

Correlations among the p IVs (i.e., psychosexual functioning, pros, cons, condom self-efficacy, and stage, all at the first time point) are given in Table 10.1. This set makes up the portion of the matrix called R_{xx} used in CC calculations. None of the correlations is indicative of collinearity among the IVs because all are less than $|0.70 - 0.90|$.

In Table 10.2 we present the portion of the matrix referred to as R_{yx} in CC analyses. Notice that all the $t2$ (indicated by B at the end of variable names) variables (i.e., the DVs) are listed down the rows and the $t1$ (A) variables (i.e., IVs) are listed across the columns at the top.

In Table 10.3 we present the R_{xy} portion of the matrix used in CC analyses. This is simply the transpose of the previous matrix, where now we have the $t1$ (A) IVs listed down the rows, and the $t2$ (B) DVs listed across the columns. Thus, each row of the R_{xy} matrix is the same as a column of the R_{yx} matrix presented above. Note that values along the diagonals of R_{yx} and R_{xy}, which are the same, give 6-month test-retest reliability correlation coefficients. All of these reveal that there is reasonable stability over the relatively long span of 6 months, for each of the five variables (i.e., values are > 0.60). If a shorter time span had been used

TABLE 10.1
(R_{xx}) Pearson Correlations (Among Xs) $(N = 527)$

	Prob > |r| under H0: Rho = 0				
	PSYXA	*PROSA*	*CONSA*	*CONSEFFA*	*STAGEA*
PSYSXA	1.000	−0.018	−0.224	0.086	−0.162
		0.663	<0.0001	0.047	0.0002
PROSA	−0.018	1.000	−0.063	0.315	0.234
	0.6636		0.145	<0.0001	<0.0001
CONSA	−0.224	−0.063	1.000	−0.402	−0.299
	<0.0001	0.145		<0.0001	<0.0001
CONSEFFA	0.086	0.315	−0.402	1.000	0.503
	0.0477	<0.0001	<0.0001		<0.0001
STAGEA	−0.162	0.234	−0.299	0.503	1.000
	0.0002	<0.0001	<0.0001	<0.0001	

TABLE 10.2
(R_{yx}) Pearson Correlations (Among Ys and Xs) ($N = 527$)

| | \multicolumn{5}{c}{Prob > \|r\| under H0: Rho = 0} |
	PSYXA	PROSA	CONSA	CONSEFFA	STAGEA
PSYSXB	0.660	−0.019	−0.225	0.119	−0.085
	<0.0001	0.6621	<0.0001	0.0059	0.0499
PROSB	0.024	0.603	−0.101	0.259	0.226
	0.5736	<0.0001	0.0193	<0.0001	<0.0001
CONSB	−0.279	−0.119	0.613	−0.368	−0.293
	<0.0001	0.0059	<0.0001	<0.0001	<0.0001
CONSEFFB	0.182	0.253	−0.399	0.615	0.383
	<0.0001	<0.0001	<0.0001	<0.0001	<0.0001
STAGEB	−0.156	0.255	−0.245	0.484	0.670
	0.0003	<0.0001	<0.0001	<0.0001	<0.0001

(e.g., 2 weeks), these values may well have been even larger and more in line with conventional standards for reliability (i.e., values > 0.70).

In Table 10.4 we present the R_{yy} portion of the matrix for use in CC analyses. This provides the intercorrelations among all of the Y or DVs, which are the same as the X or IVs except that the Ys are measured 6 months later. As with the R_{xx} portion of the matrix presented earlier, we would want to scan the correlations in the R_{yy} portion to check for collinearity within these variables (on the right, i.e., DVs). Because none of the values is > |0.70 − 0.90|, there is no reason to suspect collinearity.

TABLE 10.3
(R_{xy}) Pearson Correlations (Among Xs and Ys) ($N = 527$)

| | \multicolumn{5}{c}{Prob > \|r\| under H0: Rho = 0} |
	PSYXB	PROSB	CONSB	CONSEFFB	STAGEB
PSYSXA	0.660	0.024	−0.279	0.182	−0.156
	<0.0001	0.573	<0.0001	<0.0001	0.0003
PROSA	−0.019	0.603	−0.119	0.253	0.255
	0.6621	<0.0001	0.0059	<0.0001	<0.0001
CONSA	−0.225	−0.101	0.613	−0.399	−0.245
	<0.0001	0.0193	<0.0001	<0.0001	<0.0001
CONSEFFA	0.119	0.259	−0.368	0.615	0.484
	0.0059	<0.0001	<0.0001	<0.0001	<0.0001
STAGEA	−.085	0.226	−0.293	0.383	0.670
	0.0499	<0.0001	<0.0001	<0.0001	<0.0001

TABLE 10.4

(R_{yy}) Pearson Correlations (Among Ys) ($N = 527$)

		Prob > |r| under H0: Rho = 0			
	PSYXB	*PROSB*	*CONSB*	*CONSEFFB*	*STAGEB*
PSYSXB	1.000	0.058	−0.320	0.239	−0.103
		0.1806	<0.0001	<0.0001	0.0177
PROSB	0.058	1.000	−0.169	0.361	0.263
	0.1806		<0.0001	<0.0001	<0.0001
CONSB	−0.320	−0.169	1.000	−0.489	−0.315
	<0.0001	<0.0001		<0.0001	<0.0001
CONSEFFB	0.239	0.361	−0.489	1.000	0.447
	<0.0001	<0.0001	<0.0001		<0.0001
STAGEB	−0.103	0.263	−0.315	0.447	1.000
	0.0177	<0.0001	<0.0001	<0.0001	

Each of these four portions of the larger R_{cc} matrix is thus ready to be used in CC analyses, applying equation 1 where:

$$R_{cc} = Ryy^{-1}Ryx\ Rxx^{-1}Rxy$$

A Macro-Level Assessment of CC

The macro-level assessment in Table 10.5 reveals a small Wilks's lambda (0.11) and a large $F(25, 1922) = 63.23$, $p < 0.0001$. A multivariate effect size can easily be calculated by subtracting Wilks's lambda from 1 to yield $\eta^2 = 1 - 0.11 = 0.89$. This is very large by most standards, although in this case it represents a form of reliability coefficient for the whole set of linear combinations across a 6-month period. This indicates an impressive degree of stability from the initial time period to a follow-up assessment 6 months later.

TABLE 10.5

Macro-Level Assessment of Canonical Correlation Example

The CANCORR Procedure Multivariate Statistics and F Approximations
S = 5 M = −0.5 N = 257.5

Statistic	Value	F-Value	Num DF	Den DF	Prob. > F
Wilks' Lambda	0.10757	63.23	25	1922.1	<0.0001
Pillai's Trace	1.66440	51.99	25	2605	<0.0001
Hotteling-Lawley Trace	3.15812	65.16	25	1259.6	<0.0001
Roy's GCR	1.39731	145.60	5	521	<0.0001

Mid-Level Assessment of the CCs Among the Pairs of Canonical Variates

Table 10.6 provides macro-level results from our CC example. Given that there are five variables on each side, there are five pairs of linear combinations formed, with five corresponding canonical correlations. The canonical correlations range from 0.33 to 0.76, and all are significantly different from zero (see test of H0 in Table 10.6).

The values in the fourth column of the eigenvalues table give the proportion of the total shared variance (i.e., $1 -$ Wilks's lambda $= \eta^2$) attributed to each pair of canonical variates. As expected, the first pair is associated with the largest proportion (i.e., 0.44), whereas the fifth and last pair has a much smaller proportion (i.e., 0.04). These proportion values should add up to approximately 1.0. Thus, they are not interpreted as R^2-like values, but rather what proportion of the global shared variance between sides (i.e., $\eta^2 = 0.89$) can be attributed to each canonical correlation between pairs of canonical variates.

TABLE 10.6
Mid-Level Assessment of Canonical Correlation Example

	Canonical Correlation	Adjusted Canonical Correlation	Approximate Standard Error	Squared Canonical Correlation
		Canonical Correlation Analysis		
1	0.763457	0.756248	0.018188	0.582866
2	0.707045	0.705164	0.021805	0.499913
3	0.549183	0.544409	0.030452	0.301602
4	0.417480	0.414530	0.036003	0.174290
5	0.325161		0.038992	0.105730

Eigenvalues of Inv(E)*H = CanRsq/(1-CanRsq)

	Eigenvalue	Difference	Proportion	Cumulative
1	1.3973	0.3977	0.4425	0.4425
2	0.9997	0.5678	0.3165	0.7590
3	0.4318	0.2208	0.1367	0.8957
4	0.2111	0.0928	0.0668	0.9626
5	0.1182		0.0374	1.0000

Test of H0: The canonical correlations in the current row and all that follow are zero

	Likelihood Ratio	Approximate F-Value	Num. DF	Den. DF	Prob. > F
1	0.10757	63.23	25	1922.1	<0.0001
2	0.25789	55.24	16	1583.2	<0.0001
3	0.51570	43.89	9	1263.3	<0.0001
4	0.73840	42.57	4	1040	<0.0001
5	0.89427	61.60	1	521	<0.0001

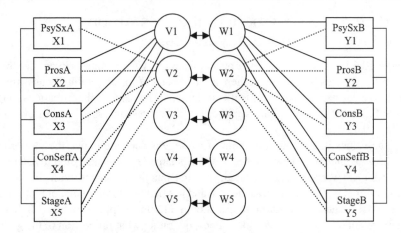

FIG. 10.3. Depiction of canonical correlation with PsySx, Pros, Cons, ConSeff, and Stage measured at times A and B, 6 months apart. The circles, labeled V1 and W1, respectively, represent the linear combinations or canonical variates for the variables on the left and the variables on the right. Lines connecting the Xs to the Vs and the Ys to the Ws represent loadings for the first two main pairs of canonical variates. Two-way arrows linking the Vs and Ws indicate canonical correlations between pairs of canonical variates.

Though all pairs are significant, we may only want to interpret the first one or two pairs that explain the bulk of the shared variance. Figure 10.3 depicts our canonical correlation example with lines for the loadings shown for only the first two pairs of canonical variates.

Micro-Level Assessment: Canonical Loadings for Both the IVs and DVs

Table 10.7 presents micro-level results for our CC example. Canonical loadings for each variable on their respective canonical variates (i.e., IVSi or DVSi) are interpreted as correlations. Values $> | 0.30 |$ reveal variables that are closely linked with the underlying canonical variate or dimension. For the first canonical variate for the Xs (i.e., IVS1), the variable that correlates most strongly is condom self-efficacy (0.82), followed closely by stage (0.78). Cons correlated -0.64 with the IVS1 and pros has a loading of 0.47. Thus, this first IV variate is associated with condom self-efficacy and a high (e.g., action or maintenance) stage of condom use. It also has something to do with perceiving relatively few cons or disadvantages to condom use and somewhat high levels of pros or advantages to using condoms. The second canonical variate is mainly concerned with psychosexual functioning (0.91), with some inverse relationship with stage (-0.38) and cons (-0.37) of condom use. Loadings for time 2 (see values for DVSi in the lower portion of

TABLE 10.7
Micro-Level Assessment of Canonical Correlation Example

Canonical Structure Correlations Between the Time 1 TTM & MMOHR
Variables and Their Canonical Variables

	IVS1 (V1)	IVS2 (V2)	IVS3 (V3)	IVS4 (V4)	IVS5 (V5)
PSYSXA	0.1608	0.9099	0.2212	0.2588	0.1740
PROSA	0.4695	−0.2714	0.8333	−0.0668	−0.0841
CONSA	−0.6379	−0.3745	0.2162	0.6360	0.0392
CONSEFFA	0.8228	−0.0028	−0.1150	0.2609	−0.4916
STAGEA	0.7813	−0.3806	−0.2297	0.1411	0.4147

Correlations Between the Time 2 TTM & MMOHR Variables and
Their Canonical Variables

	DVS1 (W1)	DVS2 (W2)	DVS3 (W3)	DVS4 (W4)	DVS5 (W5)
PSYSXB	0.2124	0.8770	0.1920	0.3195	0.2165
PROSB	0.4901	−0.1990	0.8439	−0.0573	−0.0688
CONSB	−0.6910	−0.4176	0.1347	0.5699	−0.0728
CONSEFFB	0.8093	0.1542	−0.0373	0.1757	−0.5375
STAGEB	0.7972	−0.4178	−0.2091	0.1975	0.3273

Table 10.7) parallel those for time 1 in terms of which variables are associated with which canonical variates.

Micro-Level Assessment of Redundancy: Variables on One Side and Canonical Variates on the Other Side

Table 10.8 provides redundancy coefficients, which entail correlations between a variable on one side with a canonical variate on the other side. These values are not as large as the original canonical loadings because they link time 1 variables with time 2 variates. Still, these include some relatively large values, in many cases paralleling those found within a side but with slightly smaller values. Because redundancy indices can be cumbersome to interpret, it is helpful to consider follow-up MRs to further investigate the pattern of relationships among the time 1 and time 2 variables.

Follow-Up MRs, One for Each DV, to Attempt to Examine the Directional Ordering of the Variables

Table 10.9 presents results from the first follow-up MR. This first MR reveals that psychosexual functioning, pros, cons, and condom self-efficacy are significantly related to stage of condom use 6 months later: $R^2 = 0.30$, $F(4,522) = 54.59$, $p < 0.0001$.

TABLE 10.8

Redundancy Assessment for Canonical Correlation Example

Correlations Between the Time 1 TTM & MMOHR Variables and
the Canonical Variates of the Time 2 TTM & MMOHR Variables

	DVS1 (W1)	DVS2 (W2)	DVS3 (W3)	DVS4 (W4)	DVS5 (W5)
PSYSXA	0.1228	0.6434	0.1215	0.1080	0.0566
PROSA	0.3584	−0.1919	0.4576	−0.0279	−0.0273
CONSA	−0.4870	−0.2648	0.1187	0.2655	0.0128
CONSEFFA	0.6282	−0.0020	−0.0632	0.1089	−0.1599
STAGEA	0.5965	−0.2691	−0.1262	0.0589	0.1349

Correlations Between the Time 2 TTM & MMOHR Variables and
the Canonical Variates of the Time 1 TTM & MMOHR Variables

	IVS1 (V1)	IVS2 (V2)	IVS3 (V3)	IVS4 (V4)	IVS5 (V5)
PSYSXB	0.1622	0.6201	0.1054	0.1334	0.0704
PROSB	0.3742	−0.1407	0.4634	−0.0239	−0.0224
CONSB	−0.5275	−0.2952	0.0740	0.2379	−0.0237
CONSEFFB	0.6179	0.1090	−0.0205	0.0734	−0.1748
STAGEB	0.6087	−0.2954	−0.1148	0.0825	0.1064

Table 10.10 provides micro-level results for the MR with STAGEB as the DF. All variables significantly predict stage (see t-values and associated p-values, all < 0.01). Findings suggest that stage may well be a relevant *outcome* variable, with other variables as potential predictors or causal agents.

Tables 10.11 and 10.12, respectively, present macro-level and micro-level results for the second follow-up MR with PSYSXB as the DV. Notice that relatively little variance is shared (i.e., $R^2 = 0.09$) between psychosexual functioning and

TABLE 10.9

Macro-Level Results for First Follow-Up MR: DV = STAGEB

The REG Procedure: Dependent Variable: STAGEB

Analysis of Variance

Source	df	Sum of Squares	Mean Square	F-Value	Prob. > F
Model	4	296.0212	74.0053	54.59	<0.0001
Error	522	707.5992	1.3555		
Corrected total	526	1003.6204			
Root MSE	1.16428			R-Square	0.2950
Dep. Mean	2.43643			Adjusted R^2	0.2896
Coeff Var	47.78637				

TABLE 10.10

Micro-Level Results for First Follow-Up MR: DV = STAGEB

| | | Parameter Estimates | | | | |
Variable	DF	Parameter Estimate	Standard Error	t-Value	Prob. > |t|	Standardized Estimate (β)
Intercept	1	2.299	0.417	5.50	<0.0001	0
PSYSXA	1	−0.393	0.068	−5.76	<0.0001	−0.217
PROSA	1	0.162	0.056	2.88	0.0042	0.111
CONSA	1	−0.182	0.063	−2.88	0.0041	−0.118
CONSEFFA		0.446	0.045	9.92	<0.0001	0.419

TABLE 10.11

Macro-Level Results for Second Follow-Up MR: DV = PSYSXB

The REG Procedure: Dependent Variable: PSYSXB

Analysis of Variance

Source	df	Sum of Squares	Mean Square	F-Value	Prob. > F
Model	4	26.586	6.646	12.92	<0.0001
Error	522	268.618	0.514		
Corrected total	526	295.20535			
Root MSE	0.71735			R-Square	0.0901
Dep. Mean	4.00565			Adjusted R^2	0.0831
Coeff Var	17.90850				

TABLE 10.12

Micro-Level Results for Second Follow-Up MR: DV = PSYSXB

| | | Parameter Estimates | | | | |
Variable	DF	Parameter Estimate	Standard Error	t-Value	Prob. > |t|	Standardized Estimate (β)
Intercept	1	4.527	0.176	25.68	<0.0001	0.000
PROSA	1	−0.021	0.034	−0.63	0.5302	−0.027
CONSA	1	−0.195	0.038	−5.10	<0.0001	−0.235
CONSEFFA	1	0.084	0.030	2.79	0.0054	0.146
STAGEA	1	−0.123	0.027	−4.56	<0.0001	−0.222

TABLE 10.13
Macro-Level Results for Third Follow-Up MR: DV = PROSB

The REG Procedure: Dependent Variable: PROSB

Analysis of Variance

Source	df	Sum of Squares	Mean Square	F-Value	Prob. > F
Model	4	27.849	6.962	11.55	<0.0001
Error	522	314.633	0.602		
Corrected total	526	342.483			
Root MSE	0.77637			R-Square	0.0813
Dep. Mean	4.06967			Adjusted R^2	0.0743
Coeff Var	19.07693				

the other four variables across six months. Further, one of the predictors, pros, does not significantly predict psychosexual functioning. These findings suggest that psychosexual functioning most likely is not an *outcome* variable, but if regression coefficients going from psychosexual functioning at time 1 to other variables at time 2 are significant, it may be a good predictor or potentially causal variable.

Macro-level and micro-level results from the third follow-up MR, with PROSB as the outcome, are presented in Tables 10.13 and 10.14, respectively. These MR results are not impressive with only 8% shared variance between the set of predictors and PROSB 6 months later. Further, there are two nonsignificant predictors (i.e., psychosexual functioning and cons are not significantly related to pros). As with the previous MR, this suggests that pros is most likely not a meaningful outcome or at least that there is no evidence that psychosexual functioning and cons precede pros.

TABLE 10.14
Micro-Level Results for Third Follow-Up MR: DV = PROSB

Parameter Estimates

Variable	DF	Parameter Estimate	Standard Error	t-Value	Prob. > |t|	Standardized Estimate (β)
Intercept	1	3.255	0.270	12.02	<.0001	0.000
PSYSXA	1	0.039	0.047	0.83	0.4070	0.037
CONSA	1	0.025	0.042	0.59	0.5576	0.027
CONSEFFA	1	0.121	0.031	3.82	0.0002	0.196
STAGEA	1	0.085	0.030	2.80	0.0052	0.142

TABLE 10.15
Macro-Level Results for Fourth Follow-Up MR: DV = CONSB

The REG Procedure: Dependent Variable: CONSB

Analysis of Variance

Source	df	Sum of Squares	Mean Square	F-Value	Prob. > F
Model	4	87.168	21.792	39.74	<0.0001
Error	522	286.237	0.548		
Corrected total	526	373.405			
Root MSE	0.74050			R-Square	0.2334
Dep. Mean	2.05155			Adjusted R^2	0.2276
Coeff Var	36.09488				

Tables 10.15 and 10.16 present macro-level and micro-level results, respectively, for the fourth follow-up MR, with CONSB as the DV. There is a reasonable proportion of shared variance (i.e., $R^2 = 0.23$: $F(4,522) = 39.74, p < 0.0001$) between cons at $t2$ and the other variables at $t1$, but pros is not a significant predictor. These results suggest that cons may serve as an outcome, with psychosexual functioning, condom self-efficacy, and stage potentially serving as causal predictors of cons measured 6 months later.

Still, it is worth holding back on this speculation until viewing the results from the last MR where condom self-efficacy is hypothesized as an outcome and the other variables are posited as predictors.

Tables 10.17 and 10.18 present the follow-up MR results for the fifth DV, CONSEFFB. The macro-level MR results reveal substantial shared variance (i.e., $R^2 = 0.29$: $F(4,522) = 53.98, p < 0.0001$ between the IVs and condom

TABLE 10.16
Micro-Level Results for Fourth Follow-Up MR: DV = CONSB

Parameter Estimates

Variable	DF	Parameter Estimate	Standard Error	t-Value	Prob. > |t|	Standardized Estimate (β)
Intercept	1	4.184	0.225	18.60	<.0001	0.000
PSYSXA	1	−0.327	0.043	−7.49	<.0001	−0.296
PROSA	1	−0.000	0.035	−0.01	0.9918	−0.000
CONSEFFA	1	−0.148	0.032	−4.91	<.0001	−0.228
STAGEA	1	−0.141	0.028	−4.94	<.0001	−0.226

TABLE 10.17
Macro-Level Results for Fifth Follow-Up MR: DV = CONSEFFB

The REG Procedure: Dependent Variable: CONSEFFB

Analysis of Variance

Source	df	Sum of Squares	Mean Square	F-Value	Prob. > F
Model	4	204.005	51.001	53.98	<.0001
Error	522	493.193	0.944		
Corrected total	526	697.198			
Root MSE	0.97202			R-Square	0.2926
Dep. Mean	3.51423			Adjusted R^2	0.2872
Coeff Var	27.65943				

TABLE 10.18
Micro-Level Results for Fifth Follow-Up MR: DV = CONSEFFB

Parameter Estimates

Variable	DF	Parameter Estimate	Standard Error	t-Value	Prob. > |t|	Standardized Estimate (β)
Intercept	1	1.779	0.359	4.95	<0.0001	0.000
PSYSXA	1	0.264	0.058	4.49	<0.0001	0.175
PROSA	1	0.207	0.045	4.52	<0.0001	0.171
CONSA	1	−0.334	0.051	−6.48	<0.0001	−0.261
STAGEA	1	0.250	0.034	7.19	<0.0001	0.293

self-efficacy, with all predictors significantly related to the outcome. This provides some evidence that condom self-efficacy may well serve as an outcome variable with the remaining variables (i.e., psychosexual functioning, pros, cons, and stage) serving as potentially causal predictors.

Given all the MR results, it is conceivable that both condom self-efficacy and stage are mediators or outcomes with the other variables serving as potential causal predictors.

SUMMARY

A summary of the multiplicity, background, central and interpretation themes for CC is presented in Table 10.19.

TABLE 10.19
Multiplicity, Background, Central, and Interpretation Themes Applied
to Canonical Correlation

Themes	Canonical Correlation
Multiplicity themes (Note: + means multiplicity of theme pertains)	+*Theory, hypotheses, and empirical research* +*Controls*: experimental design, select sample +*Time points*: IVs and/or DV +*Samples*: cross-validate if possible +*Measurements*: +IVs, + DVs
Background themes	*Sample data*: random selection is preferred *Measures*: multiple (continuous) IVs and DVs *Assumptions*: normality, linearity, homoscedasticity *Methods*: inferential with assumptions met
Central themes	*Variance*: in DVs shared by IVs *Covariance*: between DV and IVs and within IVs and DVs *Ratio*: covariance between X and Y / covariance within Xs and Ys
Interpretation themes	*Macro*: omnibus χ^2 or F-test, ES $= \eta^2$ *Mid*: F-tests for canonical correlation *Micro*: canonical weights (standardized or loadings),
(Questions to ask)	Redundancy analyses, and follow-up MRs Is there significant shared variance between IVs and DVs? Do pairs of canonical variates significantly correlate? Do variables correlate with their canonical variates? Do variables correlate with variates on the other side? Which DVs are significantly predicted with set of IVs? Is there little/no collinearity among variables within a side? All variables reliable? Assumptions met? Can results be generalized beyond study?

REFERENCES

Campbell, K. T., & Taylor, D. L. (1996). Canonical correlation analysis as a general linear model: A heuristic lesson for teachers and students. *Journal of Experimental Education, 64*, 157–171.

Cohen, J. (1988). *Statistical power analysis for the behavioral sciences.* San Diego, CA: Academic Press.

Cohen, J., Cohen, P., West, S. G., & Aiken, L. S. (2003). *Applied multiple regression/correlation analysis for behavioral sciences* (3rd ed.: Chapter 16, pp. 608–628). Mahwah, NJ: Lawrence Erlbaum Associates.

Fan, X. (1997). Canonical correlation analysis and structural equation modeling: What do they have in common? *Structural Equation Modeling, 4*, 65–79.

Harlow, L. L., Quina, K., Morokoff, P. J., Rose, J. S., & Grimley, D. (1993). HIV risk in women: A multifaceted model. *Journal of Applied Biobehavioral Research, 1*, 3–38.

Prochaska, J. O., Velicer, W. F., Rossi, J. S., Goldstein, M. G., Marcus, B. H., Rakowski, W., Fiore, C., Harlow, L. L., Redding, C. A., Rosenbloom, D., & Rossi, S. R. (1994). Stages of change and decisional balance for 12 problem behaviors. *Health Psychology, 13*, 39–46.

Tabachnick, B. G., & Fidell, L. S. (2001). *Using multivariate statistics* (4th ed.: Chapter 6, pp. 177–218). Boston: Allyn and Bacon.

Takane, Y., & Hwang, H. (2002). Generalized constrained canonical correlation analysis. *Multivariate Behavioral Research, 37,* 163–195.

Thompson, B. (2000). Canonical correlation analysis. In L. G. Grimm & P. R. Yarnold (Eds.), *Reading and understanding more multivariate statistics* (pp. 285–316). Washington, DC: American Psychological Association.

Thorndike, R. M. (2000). Canonical correlation analysis. In H. E. A. Tinsley, & S. D. Brown (Eds.). *Handbook of applied multivariate statistics and mathematical modeling* (pp. 237–263). San Diego, CA: Academic Press, Inc.

11

Principal Components and Factor Analysis

Themes Applied to Principal Components and Factor Analysis (PCA, FA)

PCA and FA are exploratory multivariate methods that delineate the underlying dimensions in a large set of variables or individuals. Although we consider them multivariate methods, as they indeed handle multiple variables, both methods analyze only a single set of variables. Unlike the other methods discussed in this book, there is not the usual distinction between independent and dependent variables. Still, one of our central themes in multivariate methods is that of explaining the variance and covariance within and across sets of variables. To maintain this pervasive theme, we can consider the dimensions as a set of underlying independent variables (IVs) from which the actual measured (dependent) variables (DVs) emanate. We now elucidate how the 10 questions and themes relate to both PCA and FA.

WHAT ARE PCA AND FA AND HOW ARE THEY SIMILAR TO AND DIFFERENT FROM OTHER METHODS?

PCA and FA are similar in the kinds of data that are analyzed and the conclusions drawn from these analyses. They differ somewhat in the nature of the research questions that are asked and in how they address the variance in the variables. When the goal is to redistribute the variance in a large set of correlated variables to a smaller set of orthogonal dimensions, then PCA is appropriate (Velicer & Jackson, 1990). When the focus is on identifying a set of theoretical dimensions that explain the shared common variance in a set of variables, FA can be used (e.g., Gorsuch, 1983; McDonald, 1985). Both PCA and FA allow us to examine

199

a single set of continuous variables and determine the number and nature of the underlying dimensions that organize these variables. We are, in essence, trying to find a few cogent dimensions that pull together the nature of the variables. PCA and FA locate these dimensions by noting which variables are interrelated. A main difference is that PCA uses all the variance in the variables and treats it as true variance when finding the underlying dimensions or components. FA recognizes that there is measurement error or unique variance in the variables that should be separated from the true variance or factor variance, before finding the underlying dimensions or factors. PCA is more mathematically precise. FA is more conceptually realistic. Both PCA and FA solutions can be rotated to increase interpretability. As we see later in the chapter, the two major rotation methods are Varimax (orthogonal uncorrelated) and oblique (correlated; e.g., Promax).

PCA and FA differ from most multivariate methods in that only a single set of measured variables is analyzed. PCA and FA are similar to other correlation methods that focus on the nature of the relationship among variables [e.g., multiple regression (MR), canonical correlation (CC)]. In contrast to group-difference methods [e.g., analysis of covariance (ANCOVA), multivariate analysis of variance (MANOVA)], PCA and FA do not focus on the means for a set of variables. With PCA and FA, as with several other methods [e.g., MR, discriminant function analysis (DFA), logistic regression (LR), CC], we are much more interested in

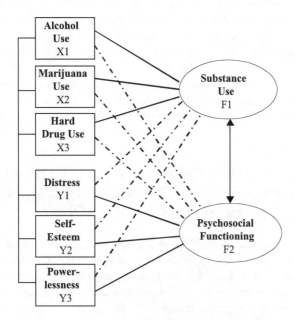

FIG. 11.1. PCA-FA with two correlated dimensions, each with three main (boldfaced) loadings and each with three inconsequential (dashed-line) loadings.

interpretable weights that link variables to underlying dimensions or linear combinations.

Figure 11.1 depicts an example of PCA-FA with two correlated dimensions: substance use and psychosocial functioning. Variables load highly on their respective dimensions, with minor loadings on the other dimension. Thus, alcohol, marijuana, and hard drug use would have high loadings on the substance use dimensions, whereas distress, self-esteem, and powerlessness would have high loadings on the psychosocial functioning dimension.

WHEN ARE PCA AND FA USED AND WHAT RESEARCH QUESTIONS CAN THEY ADDRESS?

Three main uses are offered for PCA and FA. Although both PCA and FA can be applied to all three uses, it is probably true that the ordering forms a continuum from PCA being most preferable for the first use up through FA as the best choice for the third use. That is, PCA, which is mathematically elegant, is often selected for simple orthogonal transformations of the original variables. In contrast, FA, which is conceptually oriented, is usually the method of choice for assessing the nature of the common factor variance while acknowledging the presence of uniqueness or error variance within the variables. The three basic uses are:

a. **PCA (or to some degree FA) can be used to transform a set of correlated variables into the same number of uncorrelated linear combinations or components.** These newly formed components include all the original variance in the variables, with the first component claiming most of the variance, and the remaining ones taking less and less of the variance. In effect, PCA retains all the information from the original variables while making the new components completely orthogonal, and thus more mathematically viable. There is no guarantee, however, that these mathematically elegant and orthogonal components will be conceptually interpretable. Still, these components can be used in other analyses such as MR or MANOVA to avoid possible collinearity problems.

b. **PCA or FA can be used to reduce a large set of correlated variables to a few orthogonal underlying dimensions.** These dimensions can then be rotated further, either orthogonally or obliquely (discussed later), to improve interpretation. For example, a researcher may be interested in reducing information from a 100-item inventory to a set of 10 underlying dimensions that explain much of the variance in the original variables. FA would recognize that there was most likely some measurement error or uniqueness in each item that is not analyzed when forming the dimensions or factors. The factors would involve only the variance in each item that overlaps with the other items.

c. **FA (and PCA, potentially) can be used for theory testing** to assess the conceptual nature of underlying dimensions in a set of variables. This usually involves having strong theory to suggest the nature of the variables and underlying dimensions. For example, the 12 subscales of the Wechsler intelligence tests are often delineated into verbal and performance dimensions.

WHAT ARE THE MAIN MULTIPLICITY THEMES FOR PCA AND FA?

There are several multiplicity themes that apply to PCA and FA. Even though these methods are often used in an exploratory manner, it is important to consider multiple previous theories or empirical studies that could inform the analysis. For example, theories abound today on the number and nature of dimensions underlying intelligence. Whereas initial theories (e.g., Spearman, 1904) suggested that intelligence could be described by a single, general factor, others suggest there are at least two (e.g., verbal and performance: Wechsler, 1975) or even multiple dimensions (e.g., Gardner, 1999; Matthews, 1988).

Another multiplicity theme concerns the variables. In both PCA and FA, we begin with multiple continuous measures, often viewed as DVs, and posit a smaller set of one or more (often) latent, independent dimensions that explain the correlation among the variables. We also most likely would want a large sample size, although guidelines vary on how large. Some (e.g., Comrey & Lee, 1992) focus on the recommended total size needed to achieve stability of results, with samples of at least 200 to 300 being preferred. Other methods focus on the ratio of participants to number of variables (e.g., MR), though this does not have much evidence with PCA or FA (Guadagnoli & Velicer, 1988). Finally, recent researchers (e.g., Guadagnoli & Velicer, 1988) suggest that a smaller sample size (e.g., 100 to 200) may be adequate if the dimensions are highly saturated. This would occur if the three to six variables that marked each factor had rather high loadings (e.g., at least | 0.50 | or even | 0.70 | or higher).

WHAT ARE THE MAIN BACKGROUND THEMES APPLIED TO PCA AND FA?

With both PCA and FA, background themes would include an examination of correlations, but not necessarily the means for a set of variables. Correlations should be greater than | 0.30 | among variables within a dimension. Correlations among variables from different dimensions should be close to zero if dimensions are expected to be orthogonal (i.e., uncorrelated), though some nonzero correlations are acceptable, particularly with dimensions that are expected to be oblique (i.e., correlated). The issue of collinearity, although not as much of a problem as with other methods, should still be investigated. Variables within a dimension are often viewed as similar ways of expressing the same dimension and thus can exhibit substantial correlation (e.g., | 0.30 to 0.70 |). However, if correlation exceeds | 0.90 |, there could be problems associated with collinearity (e.g., instability of the weights or loadings). If collinearity is suspected, consider collapsing the two variables involved into an averaged or summed composite or even dropping one of the variables.

As with most multivariate methods, we would like to have access to a large ($N \times p$) data matrix with multiple continuous variables. Unlike many methods, there would be less emphasis on meeting statistical assumptions, particularly when making only descriptive summaries of the data. Certainly, inferences beyond a specific sample would be strengthened when meeting linear model assumptions (i.e., normality, linearity, and homoscedasticity) in a large and relevant sample. Finally, the reliability of each variable is also a concern. Ideally, we would like internal consistency coefficients to be 0.70 or higher, but test–retest reliability, especially over long time periods (e.g., 6 to 12 months) may not be quite as high.

WHAT IS THE STATISTICAL MODEL THAT IS TESTED WITH PCA AND FA?

For PCA, we model the underlying linear combination or component, V, as a function of the original X variables and eigenvector weights:

$$V = XB \tag{11.1}$$

where V is a linear combination or component, X is a continuous variable, and B is a matrix of eigenvector weights. The variance covariance matrix of the components would be a diagonal matrix with eigenvalues (i.e., variances) of the linear combinations along the diagonals and zeroes elsewhere due to orthogonality of the components. This diagonal matrix can be described in matrix form as:

$$S_C = B'S_X B \tag{11.2}$$

where S_C is a (q by q) matrix of variances and covariances among the q components, B is a (p by q) matrix of eigenvector weights, B' is the transpose of the B matrix of eigenvector weights, and S_X is a (p by p) matrix of variances and covariances among the p original X variables. Equation 11.2 highlights the relationship among the eigenvalues and eigenvectors and the original variables. It states that when we pre- and post-multiply the original variance-covariance matrix for the X variables by the matrix of eigenvector weights, we will get a diagonal matrix with the variances of the new components along the diagonal. The goal in PCA is to choose the eigenvector weights so that much of the variance from the variables is preserved in the first few components. Note that all the variance in the variables is retained and redistributed in PCA.

For FA, the underlying dimension is not modeled, but rather the original X variable is modeled as a function of the underlying dimension times a (factor loading) weight plus some uniqueness:

$$X = LF + E \qquad (11.3)$$

where X is a (p by 1) vector of variables, L is a (p by q) matrix of factor loadings for the p continuous variables and the q underlying factors, F is a (q by 1) vector of factors, and E is a (p by 1) vector of uniquenesses for the p continuous X variables. The variance covariance matrix of the X variables is modeled as:

$$S_X = L\Phi L' + \Theta \qquad (11.4)$$

where S_X is a (p by p) matrix of variances and covariances among the original X variables, L is the (p by q) matrix of factor loadings, Φ is a (q by q) matrix of variances and covariances among the factors, and Θ is a (p by p) matrix of variances and covariances among the p uniquenesses (or measurement errors) for the original variables. The goal in FA is to find the parameters (i.e., factor loadings, factor variances and covariances, and uniquenesses) that will reproduce the original variance-covariance matrix for the original X variables as closely as possible.

HOW DO CENTRAL THEMES OF VARIANCE, COVARIANCE, AND LINEAR COMBINATIONS APPLY TO PCA AND FA?

As we saw with the descriptions of the equations for PCA and FA, variance is examined differently for the two methods. In PCA, we examine all the variance and do not even consider the possibility of error variance in the variables. Thus, PCA uses the matrix of correlations among the variables as the initial starting point for analysis. The p standardized variances (i.e., 1s) along the diagonal are redistributed among the new components. This method assumes that the variables are perfectly reliable and that all the variance in the variables is worth retaining.

In FA, we recognize that each variable has a portion of true-score variance (e.g., Lord & Novick, 1968) as well as some portion that is not shared with the other variables loading on a factor. The focus of FA is on the portion of the variance in a variable that is shared in common with the other variables and thus is called common factor variance. In FA, then, we use a matrix of correlations as the starting point, except that instead of 1s along the diagonal, we insert *communalities*, which are estimates of the shared variance between a specific variable and all the remaining variables. Remembering back to MR, we see that a squared multiple correlation (SMC or R^2) between a variable and the remaining variables provides a measure of shared variance. Another estimate of communality is the absolute value of the largest correlation within a factor (Gorsuch, 1983). These estimates values are often inserted along the diagonal in FA to reflect the fact that we are analyzing only the portion of variance in the original variables that is held in common among the variables. The diagonal matrix of unique or error variance holds the remaining variance so that when adding this matrix to the correlation matrix with SMCs along the diagonal we get the full R matrix of correlations among the variables (i.e., with 1s along the diagonals).

Covariance plays a central role in that variables must have some covariance if there are underlying dimensions that explain the relatedness among the variables. One rule of thumb is to make sure there are at least several correlations of at least | 0.30 | or more to ensure the presence of one or more dimensions. If all the variables were completely orthogonal (i.e., correlations were equal to zero), it would not be possible to describe the set of p variables with a smaller set of q dimensions.

Finally, linear combinations are viewed differently between PCA and FA. In PCA, the linear combination of interest is the new component score that is a function of the original variables and a set of eigenvector weights. In FA, the linear combination that we focus on is the original X variable, which is seen as a weighted function of an underlying factor plus some uniqueness or measurement error.

WHAT ARE THE MAIN THEMES NEEDED
TO INTERPRET PCA AND FA RESULTS
AT A MACRO-LEVEL?

In contrast to the other multivariate methods we discussed, PCA does not usually have a significance test associated with it. When using FA, a maximum likelihood test is occasionally used to test for the number of factors (see below). However, the test is often too sensitive, suggesting too many factors to retain. Thus, it is not often used for exploratory FA. It is used with confirmatory FA and other structural equation modeling methods, but it is a topic not addressed here.

PCA and FA usually focus on one or more of the following to address macro-level assessment:

a. **The percentage of variance in the variables that is accounted for by the factors** is a useful index for assessing the viability of the factors. While the dimensions may not be expected to explain all the variation and covariation among the variables, it would be reasonable to explain at least 50% or more. We get an indication of the proportion of variance explained by a dimension by forming a ratio of an eigenvalue over the sum of all the eigenvalues.

b. **The number of eigenvalues greater than 1.0** is often used as an upper-bound estimate on the number of underlying components in PCA. Guttman (1954) and Kaiser (1970) advocated the method to help in deciding on the correct number of dimensions, but the true number may well be less than this. The rationale was that the variance of a single, standardized variable would be 1.0 (e.g., consider the diagonals of a correlation matrix). If an underlying dimension were to be worth examining, it would have to have at least the same amount of variance as a single variable, but ideally it should have much more variance.

c. Another method for assessing the number of dimensions (either components or factors) is to examine when the eigenvalues appear to be dropping off to a trivial, inconsequential size. **The scree plot** (Cattell, 1966) involves a plot of the number of factors on the X axis by the values of the eigenvalues on the Y axis. The point at or before the elbow in a scree plot provides another estimation as to the number of underlying dimensions. Cattell reasoned that this plot would drop off much like the scree or rubble at the bottom of a hillside after most of the variance in a set of variables has been explained by the set of factors.

d. Two other methods have been suggested to help identify the correct number of dimensions to retain. **Velicer's (1976) minimum average partials (MAP) method**, as well as **Horn's (1965) parallel analysis method**, have been found to be fairly accurate with estimating the number of dimensions in a set of variables (e.g., Zwick & Velicer, 1986).

e. It is often important to make a **qualitative assessment of the interpretability of the factors** and relevance to theory as another indication of the usefulness of a solution.

f. Finally, it is possible to have a χ^2 **test of significance** when using maximum-likelihood factor analysis to assess whether the correct number of factors is retained; this is not commonly used.

WHAT ARE THE MAIN THEMES NEEDED TO INTERPRET PCA AND FA RESULTS AT A MICRO-LEVEL?

The main question to ask at the micro-level for both PCA and FA is this: Are the variables related to underlying dimensions?

a. Similar to several other methods (e.g., MR, DFA, LR, CC), PCA and FA **focus on weights** attached to specific variables to get a microperspective. Just as with DFA and CC, the most interpretable weight is a (component or factor) loading or structure coefficient. Unlike most applications of DFA and CC, the loadings are often rotated in PCA and FA to increase the interpretability of the dimensions. There are several kinds of rotation procedures, but the most common are Varimax, which rotates dimensions orthogonally, and oblique (e.g., Promax), which allows dimensions to be correlated. While most computer programs use the Varimax orthogonal rotation as a default option, it is often useful to consider an oblique rotation. This is especially true if we expect the dimensions to be related. In either case, we usually strive to rotate the weights so that each dimension has several variables that load highly with the remaining variables loading close to zero. This pattern is labeled a "simple structure" (Thurstone, 1935), which is strived for but not always achieved. In any structure, whether simple or not, loadings range from -1 to $+1$ and show how correlated a variable is with an underlying dimension (i.e., component or factor). For both PCA and FA, we use the same criterion as with other methods that rely on loadings; variables with loadings of $|0.30|$ or greater are interpreted as having a meaningful part on the whole dimension. We also would like to try to describe the nature of each dimension by noting the kind of variables that highly load on the components and factors. As with other methods that focus on weights, the sign attached to a loading informs us about the nature of the relationship. A positive value indicates that a variable is very similar to the underlying dimension. A negative loading suggests that the higher the score on the respective variable, the lower the score on the dimension on which the variable loads. Thus, variables could be evaluated with several guidelines (see below).

b. **Those with loadings** $\geq|0.30|$ **would be retained** as marker variables for a dimension, with ideally three or more marker variables per dimension.

c. **Variables with loadings** $<|0.30|$ **on all dimensions could be discarded.** This would not necessarily mean the variables are unreliable. It could be the variables do not have enough in common with the other variables. If this is the case, more variables addressing the same content could be included in a future study to help anchor the additional dimension.

d. **Those with loadings** $\geq|0.30|$ **on more than one dimension would be labeled as complex variables.** Complex variables most likely would be discarded because it would not be clear to which dimension the variable was describing.

e. **Variables that had positive and high loadings** would be most consistent with the direction and nature of a dimension.

f. **Those with negative and high loadings** would indicate variables that are inversely related to an underlying dimension.

WHAT ARE SOME OTHER CONSIDERATIONS OR NEXT STEPS AFTER APPLYING PCA OR FA?

PCA and FA, like CC, are exploratory procedures that usually lend themselves to descriptive conclusions, though not necessarily inferences to the larger population. After conducting a PCA or FA on a sample of data, it would be wise to consider several follow-ups.

If statistical assumptions are met and a large, representative, and ideally random sample is analyzed, then generalizations beyond the immediate sample become more credible. Lykken's (1968) emphasis on constructive replication is relevant here. Lykken argues that results from a single study are much more convincing when replicated with separate, independent samples, different items to anchor each of the major dimensions, and different methods. Thus, exploratory PCA or FA results would be more compelling if replicated in a separate sample or if the same factor structure were found using different items for each of the main constructs. Further, confirmatory methods such as confirmatory factor analysis (CFA) should be considered. CFA is a subset of structural equation modeling in which several latent factors are posited, with each of them having hypothesized loadings on several salient variables. In CFA, the number and nature of the factors is known at the beginning of the study. The goal is to assess how well the hypothesized structure fits the data. Though the topic of CFA is beyond the scope of this book, several excellent sources describe this useful methodology and the larger method of structural equation modeling (e.g., Bentler, 2000; Byrne, 2001; Loehlin, 2004; Raykov & Marcoulides, 2000; Schumacker & Lomax, 2004).

If follow-up results appear encouraging, there would be greater verisimilitude for the underlying dimensions that could be used to summarize scores on a measuring instrument or even used in a predictive framework, such as structural equation modeling.

WHAT IS AN EXAMPLE OF APPLYING PCA AND FA TO A RESEARCH QUESTION?

For this example, we examine the set of three condom use variables (i.e., pros, cons, and self-efficacy) from the transtheoretical model (e.g., Prochaska et al., 1994), as well as five MMOHR (Harlow et al., 1993) variables (psychosexual functioning, meaninglessness, stress, demoralization, and powerlessness) representing psychosocial distress. All eight variables are measured at the initial time point, $t1$. Several sets of analyses are presented: a, descriptive statistics for the p variables; b, correlations among the p variables; c, a macro- and micro-level assessment of PCA; and d, a macro- and micro-level assessment of FA.

Descriptive Statistics for the Variables

Table 11.1 presents descriptive statistics for the variables used in the PCA and FA application. Note that the three positively focused variables (i.e., pros, self-efficacy, and psychosexual functioning) all have rather high means (i.e., 3.85, 3.29, and 3.99, respectively) relative to the remaining negatively focused variables. Most of the variables are relatively normally distributed. Two slight exceptions

TABLE 11.1
Descriptive Statistics on the Variables in the PCA and FA Example

			The MEANS Procedure			
Variable	*Mean*	*S.D.*	*Min.*	*Max.*	*Skewness*	*Kurtosis*
PROSA	3.86	0.95	1.00	5.00	−1.000	0.587
CONSA	2.14	0.90	1.00	5.00	0.709	0.077
CONSEFFA	3.29	1.30	1.00	5.00	−0.305	−1.189
PSYSXA	3.99	0.76	1.00	5.00	−0.853	0.793
MELESSA	2.24	0.79	1.00	5.00	0.544	−0.187
STRESSA	2.55	0.60	1.00	4.50	0.209	−0.011
DEMORA	2.23	0.56	1.00	4.08	0.479	0.029
PWRLSSA	2.18	0.68	1.00	4.60	0.632	0.223

involve pros with some negative skewness (i.e., most people report a high level of perceived advantages of condom use), and condom self-efficacy (CONSEFFA) that has some negative kurtosis (i.e., there is a platykurtic distribution, so that there are approximately an equal number of people who report low, medium, and high levels of condom self efficacy). Still, there does not appear to be enough nonnormality to warrant making transformations of the data.

Correlations Among the p Variables

We would now want to examine a matrix of correlations among the eight variables to ensure that there were some correlations of at least | 0.30 | or more, as well as to make sure there was not high collinearity (i.e., $r > | 0.70$ to $0.90 |$). The correlation matrix shown in Table 11.2 suggests that these variables would be reasonable for both PCA and FA.

Macro- and Micro-Level Assessment of PCA

We have seen that the macro-level PCA or FA does not usually involve a significance test but rather an examination of the number and nature of the dimensions. Table 11.3 presents information on the eigenvalues for our example.

Several criteria indicate two components for the set of variables. First, there are two eigenvalues greater than 1.0. This guideline provides an approximate estimate as to the number of components underlying a set of variables (e.g., Guttman, 1954; Kaiser, 1970; Preacher & MacCallum, 2003). Second, the percentage of variance in the variables that is extracted by two dimensions is greater than 50% (i.e., 61%: see cumulative column in Table 11.3). With more than half the information in the variables explained by the two components, we have assurance that the dimensions are adequately describing the variables.

TABLE 11.2
Pearson Correlation Coefficients

	PROSA	CONSA	CONSEFFA	PSYSXA
		Prob $> \mid r \mid$ under H0 : Rho $= 0$		
PROSA	1.00000	−0.06348	0.31509	−0.01899
		0.1456	<0.0001	0.6636
CONSA	−0.06348	1.00000	−0.40206	−0.22409
	0.1456		<0.0001	<0.0001
CONSEFFA	0.31509	−0.40206	1.00000	0.08629
	<0.0001	<0.0001		0.0477
PSYSXA	−0.01899	−0.22409	0.08629	1.00000
	0.6636	<0.0001	0.0477	
MELESSA	−0.07058	0.13682	−0.08182	−0.38522
	0.1056	0.0016	0.0605	<0.0001
STRESSA	−0.03748	0.13492	−0.08081	−0.37505
	0.3906	0.0019	0.0638	<0.0001
DEMORA	−0.03119	0.20517	−0.11410	−0.41345
	0.4749	<0.0001	0.0087	<0.0001
PWRLSSA	−0.08547	0.18307	−0.11526	−0.41353
	0.0499	<0.0001	0.0081	<0.0001
	MELESSA	*STRESSA*	*DEMORA*	*PWRLSSA*
PROSA	−0.07058	−0.03748	−0.03119	−0.08547
	0.1056	0.3906	0.4749	0.0499
CONSA	0.13682	0.13492	0.20517	0.18307
	0.0016	0.0019	<0.0001	<0.0001
CONSEFFA	−0.08182	−0.08081	−0.11410	−0.11526
	0.0605	0.0638	0.0087	0.0081
PSYSXA	−0.38522	−0.37505	−0.41345	−0.41353
	<0.0001	<0.0001	<0.0001	<0.0001
MELESSA	1.00000	0.62807	0.74492	0.67889
		<0.0001	<0.0001	<0.0001
STRESSA	0.62807	1.00000	0.74902	0.64129
	<0.0001		<0.0001	<0.0001
DEMORA	0.74492	0.74902	1.00000	0.70569
	<0.0001	<0.0001		<0.0001
PWRLSSA	0.67889	0.64129	0.70569	1.00000
	<0.0001	<0.0001	<0.0001	

Figure 11.2 presents the plot of the eigenvalues (i.e., scree plot: Cattell, 1966) for these data. The eigenvalues from Table 11.3 are plotted along the vertical axis and the dimensions (up to the number of variables analyzed) are listed along the horizontal axis. The steep drop in the plot of the first two eigenvalues, followed by a shallower slope in the plot for the remaining eigenvalues also suggests that two dimensions would adequately represent the data.

TABLE 11.3
Principal Component Loadings for the Example

The FACTOR Procedure.
Initial Factor Method: Principal Components
Prior Communality Estimates: ONE
Eigenvalues of the Correlation Matrix:
Total = 8   Average = 1

	Eigenvalue	Difference	Proportion	Cumulative
1	3.44689334	1.98527664	0.4309	0.4309
2	1.46161670	0.48347860	0.1827	0.6136
3	0.97813810	0.29155964	0.1223	0.7358
4	0.68657846	0.17400935	0.0858	0.8217
5	0.51256911	0.13143969	0.0641	0.8857
6	0.38112942	0.05566134	0.0476	0.9334
7	0.32546808	0.11786128	0.0407	0.9740
8	0.20760680		0.0260	1.0000

2 factors will be retained by the NFACTOR criterion.

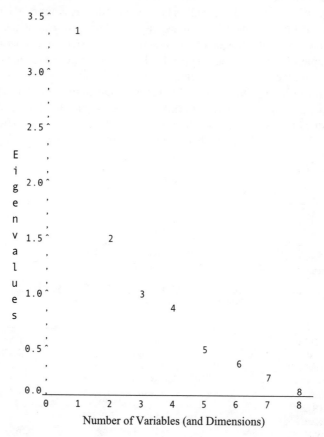

FIG. 11.2.   Scree Plot of Eigenvalues for the Example with Eight Variables.

TABLE 11.4
Micro-Assessment of PCA with Orthogonal, Varimax Rotation

Principal Components, Rotation Method: Varimax
Rotated Factor Pattern

	Factor 1	Factor 2
PROSA	0.01731	0.59637
CONSA	0.18740	−0.66556
CONSEFFA	−0.04438	0.85159
PSYSXA	−0.58151	0.11248
MELESSA	0.85518	−0.04023
STRESSA	0.84651	−0.02091
DEMORA	0.90166	−0.06988
PWRLSSA	0.84789	−0.09858

Another consideration is that the two dimensions should have theoretical relevance to justify retaining them. This is best evaluated by examining the pattern of loadings on the two retained dimensions. Table 11.4 presents component loadings that have been rotated orthogonally, assuming that the two components are uncorrelated. Table 11.5 presents component loadings that have been rotated obliquely, also providing the degree of correlation between the two dimensions. Both the orthogonal (Varimax) and oblique (Promax) solutions indicate two relatively uncorrelated (i.e., $r = -0.16$) components with near simple structure. Factor 1 has high loadings for psychosocial variables hypothesized in the MMOHR (Harlow et al., 1993). Factor 2 has high loadings for condom use variables from the

TABLE 11.5
Micro-Assessment of PCA with Oblique, Promax Rotation

Inter-Factor Correlations

	Factor 1	Factor 2
Factor 1	1.00000	−0.16024
Factor 2	−0.16024	1.00000

Principal Components, Rotation Method: Promax
Factor Structure (Correlations: loadings)

	Factor 1	Factor 2
PROSA	−0.03010	0.59298
CONSA	0.23966	−0.67860
CONSEFFA	−0.11186	0.85238
PSYSXA	−0.58861	0.15942
MELESSA	0.85568	−0.10967
STRESSA	0.84549	−0.08971
DEMORA	0.90437	−0.14300
PWRLSSA	0.85304	−0.16723

TABLE 11.6

Macro-Level Assessment of FA for the Eight-Variable Example

The FACTOR Procedure
Initial Factor Method: Principal Factors
Prior Communality Estimates: SMC

PROSA	CONSA	CONSEFFA	PSYSXA
0.11567833	0.21306340	0.24691142	0.22988046
MELESSA	*STRESSA*	*DEMORA*	*PWRLSSA*
0.60872477	0.59204055	0.71379320	0.58129199

Eigenvalues of the Reduced Correlation Matrix:
Total = 3.30138412 Average = 0.41267302

	Eigenvalue	Difference	Proportion	Cumulative
1	3.02161613	2.33134886	0.9153	0.9153
2	0.69026727	0.52423147	0.2091	1.1243
3	0.16603580	0.16993609	0.0503	1.1746
4	−.00390029	0.04850678	−.0012	1.1735
5	−.05240707	0.05349322	−.0159	1.1576
6	−.10590029	0.03200424	−.0321	1.1255
7	−.13790453	0.13851836	−.0418	1.0837
8	−.27642289		−.0837	1.0000

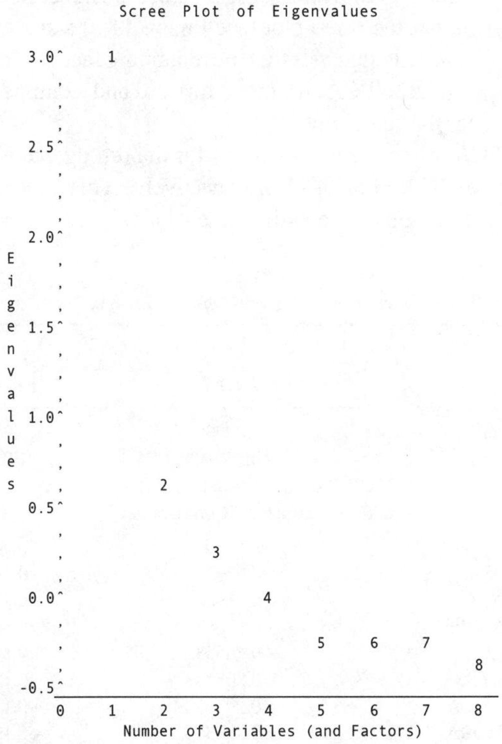

FIG. 11.3. Scree Plot for the Eight-Variable FA Example.

TABLE 11.7
Micro-Assessment of FA with Orthogonal Rotation

Rotation Method: Varimax
Rotated Factor Pattern

	Factor 1	Factor 2
PROSA	−0.01264	0.35053
CONSA	0.16242	−0.49090
CONSEFFA	−0.05429	0.60983
PSYSXA	−0.47306	0.13533
MELESSA	0.80569	−0.06856
STRESSA	0.79321	−0.05118
DEMORA	0.87755	−0.10085
PWRLSSA	0.78839	−0.13072

transtheoretical model (Prochaska et al., 1994). Thus, we could conclude that the two components have both theoretical and empirical support.

Macro- and Micro-Level Assessment of FA

While it is not as clear-cut as with PCA, there appears to be evidence for two factors with a FA of these same eight variables. Eigenvalues are not easily interpreted with FA (see Table 11.6), but the scree plot (see Figure 11.3) starts to form an elbow after the second factor. This suggests that the remaining factors would not be worth examining. Thus, similar to PCA, we move forward and examine two dimensions at a micro-level after the scree plot.

As with the PCA micro-results, loadings for the orthogonal and oblique solutions are similar (see Tables 11.7 & 11.8, respectively). This is most likely due to the relatively small correlation between the dimensions (i.e., $r = -0.23$). Compared

TABLE 11.8
Micro-Assessment of FA with Oblique, Promax Rotation

Inter-Factor Correlations

	Factor 1	Factor 2
Factor 1	1.00000	−0.23088
Factor 2	−0.23088	1.00000

The FACTOR Procedure: Rotation Method: Promax
Factor Structure (Correlations)

	Factor 1	Factor 2
PROSA	−0.05438	0.34971
CONSA	0.21984	−0.50612
CONSEFFA	−0.12667	0.61206
PSYSXA	−0.48583	0.18798
MELESSA	0.80812	−0.15927
STRESSA	0.79365	−0.14059
DEMORA	0.88331	−0.19948
PWRLSSA	0.79835	−0.21908

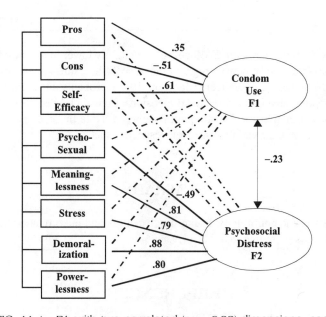

FIG. 11.4. FA with two correlated (*r* = −0.23) dimensions, each with 3+ main (boldfaced) loadings ≥| 0.30 | and 3+ inconsequential (dashed-lined) loadings <| 0.30 |

TABLE 11.9
Multiplicity, Background, Central, and Interpretation Themes Applied to PCA-FA

Themes	*Principal Components-Factor Analysis*
Multiplicity themes (Note: + means multiplicity of theme pertains)	+*Theory, hypotheses and empirical research*
	Controls: (few)
	Time points: Replicate?
	Samples: cross-validate
	+*Measurements*: +DVs, +Dimensions
Background themes	*Sample data*: random selection
	Measures: multiple continuous DVs, 1+ latent (IV) dimensions
	Assumptions: (normality, linearity, homoscedasticity)
	Methods: descriptive or inferential with theory, random sample, and assumptions met
Central themes	*Variance*: in DVs explained by dimensions
	Covariance: among DVs and dimensions (i.e., loadings)
	Ratio: Proportion of variance for dimensions
Interpretation themes (questions to ask)	*Macro*: number of dimensions
	Micro: dimension loadings
	Do dimensions explain enough variance?
	Are all variables reliable and needed?
	High correlation within dimensions?
	Low correlations across dimensions?
	3+ marker variables per dimension?
	Which variables load on each dimension?
	Assumptions met?
	Can design support causal inference?

with PCA loadings, however, FA loadings are slightly lower in magnitude for the marker variables and somewhat higher otherwise. Still, results appear comparable across PCA and FA (e.g., Velicer & Jackson, 1990), probably due to fairly reliable variables and relatively uncorrelated dimensions. Figure 11.4 depicts the loadings and factor correlation for the oblique FA solution. Note that factor loadings are given only for marker variables on their respective factors.

SUMMARY

A summary of the multiplicity, background, central, and interpretation themes for PCA and FA is presented in Table 11.9.

REFERENCES

Bentler, P. M. (2000). *EQS6: Structural equations program manual*. Encino, CA: Multivariate Software, Inc.

Byrne, B. M. (2001). *Structural equation modeling with AMOS: Basic concepts, applications, and programming*. Mahwah, NJ: Lawrence Erlbaum Associates.

Cattell, R. B. (1966). The scree test for the number of factors. *Multivariate Behavioral Research, 1*, 245–266.

Comrey, A. L., & Lee, H. B. (1992). *A first course in factor analysis* (2nd ed.). Hillsdale, NJ: Lawrence Erlbaum Associates.

Gardner, H. (1999). *Intelligence reframed: Multiple intelligences for the 21st century*. New York: Basic Books.

Gorsuch, R. L. (1983). *Factor Analysis* (2nd ed.). Hillsdale, NJ: Erlbaum.

Guadagnoli, E., & Velicer, W. F. (1988). Relation of sample size to the stability of component patterns. *Psychological Bulletin, 10*, 265–275.

Guttman, L. (1954). Some necessary conditions for common factor analysis. *Psychometrika, 19*, 149–161.

Horn, J. L. (1965). A rationale and test for the number of factors in factor analysis. *Psychometrika, 30*, 179–185.

Harlow, L. L., Quina, K., Morokoff, P. J., Rose, J. S., & Grimley, D. (1993). HIV risk in women: A multifaceted model. *Journal of Applied Biobehavioral Research, 1*, 3–38.

Kaiser, H. F. (1970). A second generation Little Jiffy. *Psychometrika, 35*, 401–415.

Loehlin, J. C. (2004). *Latent variable models: An introduction to factor, path, and structural equation analysis* (4th ed.). Mahwah, NJ: Lawrence, Erlbaum Associates.

Lord, F. M., & Novick, M. R. (1968). *Statistical theories of mental test scores*. Reading, MA: Addison-Wesley Publishing Company, Inc.

Lykken, D. T. (1968). Statistical significance in psychological research. *Psychological Bulletin, 70*, 151–159.

Matthews, D. J. (1988). Gardner's Multiple Intelligence theory: An evaluation of relevant research literature and a consideration of its application to gifted education. *Roeper Review, 11*, 100–104.

McDonald, R. P. (1985). *Factor analysis and related methods*. Hillsdale, NJ: Erlbaum.

Preacher, K. J., & MacCallum, R. C. (2003). Repairing Tom Swift's electric factor analysis machine. *Understanding Statistics, 2*, 13–43.

Prochaska, J. O., Velicer, W. F., Rossi, J. S., Goldstein, M. G., Marcus, B. H., Rakowski, W., Fiore, C., Harlow, L. L., Redding, C. A., Rosenbloom, D., & Rossi, S. R. (1994). Stages of change and decisional balance for 12 problem behaviors. *Health Psychology, 13*, 39–46.

Raykov, T., & Marcoulides, G. A. (2000). *A first course in structural equation modeling*. Mahwah, NJ: Lawrence Erlbaum Associates.

Schumacker, R. E., & Lomax, R. G. (2004). *A beginner's guide to structural equation modeling* (2nd ed.). Mahwah, NJ: Lawrence Erlbaum Associates.

Spearman, C. (1904). General intelligence, objectively measured. *American Journal of Psychology, 38*, 201–293.

Thurstone, L. L. (1935). *The vectors of the mind*. Chicago: University of Chicago Press.

Velicer, W. F. (1976). Determining the number of components from the matrix of partial correlations. *Psychometrika, 41*, 321–327.

Velicer, W. F., & Jackson, D. N. (1990). Component analysis vs. common factor analysis: Some issues in selecting an appropriate procedure. *Multivariate Behavioral Research, 25*, 1–28.

Wechsler, D. (1975). Intelligence defined and undefined: A relativistic appraisal. *American Psychologist, 30*, 135–139.

Zwick, W. R., & Velicer, W. F. (1986). Factor influencing five rules for determining the number of components to retain. *Psychological Bulletin, 99*, 432–442.

VI

Summary

12

Integration of Multivariate Methods

Themes Applied to Multivariate Methods

Consider each of the 10 themes, below, for the multivariate methods covered.

WHAT ARE THE MULTIVARIATE METHODS AND HOW ARE THEY SIMILAR AND DIFFERENT?

All seven of the multivariate methods [i.e., multiple regression (MR), analysis of covariance (ANCOVA), multivariate analysis of variance (MANOVA), discriminant function analysis (DFA), logistic regression (LR), canonical correlation (CC), principal components analysis and factor analysis (PCA-FA)] covered in this book can analyze multiple variables, taking into account other variables in the analysis. All the methods involve some form of linear combination, with some methods (e.g., DFA, CC, PCA, FA) having more than one of these. Most of the methods (i.e., MANOVA, DFA, CC, PCA, and FA) involve eigenvalues that are variances of the linear combinations.

For all seven of the methods, inferences beyond the sample analyzed are improved to the extent that assumptions (e.g., normality, linearity, and homoscedasticity) are met, but LR, PCA, and FA do not always require assumptions. The methods differ based on the nature of the variables and the focus of the research questions addressed (more discussion is presented later on research questions in section When are Multivariate Methods used and What Research Questions Can They Address? and on the nature of the variables in section What Are the Main Background Themes Applied to Methods?).

Correlational methods include MR, CC, PCA-FA, and to some degree DFA, with each of these methods focusing on weights that can be interpreted in a correlational metric. These methods focus little, if at all, on mean differences, although DFA may involve group centroids that are means of the linear combinations (i.e., discriminant functions). MR, CC, PCA, and FA use predominantly continuous variables, with DFA also including a categorical outcome in addition to continuous independent variables (IVs) with categorical IVs allowed.

Methods with one or more major categorical variables include ANCOVA, MANOVA, DFA, and LR. Whereas ANCOVA and MANOVA have one or more categorical IVs, DFA and LR have a single categorical outcome. LR also allows categorical IVs, whereas in DFA the IVs are usually continuous. There is a single continuous outcome variable in ANCOVA, with MANOVA allowing two or more continuous outcomes. The last two methods focus on mean differences between groups, whereas DFA and LR focus more on interpreting weights between a set of IVs and a single categorical outcome. These four methods (AN-COVA, MANOVA, DFA, and LR), involving one or more categorical variables, each relates one or more IVs to one or more dependent variables (DVs).

All the methods covered allow both macro- and micro-assessment of the effect (i.e., shared variance) between IVs and DVs, but the IVs in PCA and FA are underlying dimensions.

We now turn to a discussion of multivariate methods and research questions.

WHEN ARE MULTIVARIATE METHODS USED AND WHAT RESEARCH QUESTIONS CAN THEY ADDRESS?

Research questions that involve prediction can use multivariate methods of MR, DFA, LR, or CC. All these methods involve multiple predictors, with the first three methods including a single DV and the latter involving two or more DVs. For all four prediction methods, the focus is on examining the degree of relationship between the IVs and DV(s) and then interpreting weights at the micro-level.

Research questions involving group differences would most likely draw on the multivariate methods of ANCOVA or MANOVA and possibly DFA. For the former two methods, analyses focus on whether the means of the DV(s) differ between two or more groups, relative to within-group differences. DFA may focus on group centroids, but the emphasis is more likely to be on classification or weights.

PCA and FA are multivariate methods that involve a single set of measured variables plus one or more underlying dimensions (labeled components for PCA and factors for FA). The goal of these methods is to describe the correlational structure among a set of variables with a few central components or factors. PCA and FA differ in the variance that is analyzed and whether measurement error is recognized. PCA analyzes all the variance in the measures, ignoring any mention of measurement error. FA analyzes only the common variance among the variables, separating out the unique or measurement error variance.

We turn now to a discussion of the multivariate themes across the methods.

WHAT ARE THE MAIN MULTIPLICITY THEMES FOR METHODS?

Table 12.1 presents an overview of the multiplicity themes for the multivariate methods addressed in this book. MR, ANCOVA, MANOVA, and DFA would most likely draw on multiple theories and empirical studies to motivate one or more hypotheses. LR, CC, PCA, and FA may or may not emphasize theories, empirical studies, or hypotheses, depending on whether there was a more rigorous inferential or, conversely, a more exploratory descriptive focus, respectively.

Most of the methods (MR, ANCOVA, MANOVA, DFA, LR, and CC) could involve multiple time points and controls, but this is less likely to be true of PCA and FA.

Four of the methods involve grouping variables, with ANCOVA and MANOVA each having IV(s) with two or more groups, and DFA and LR each having a single DV with two or more groups or categories. All the methods involve IVs, with MR, DFA, LR, and CC having two or more IVs. ANCOVA and MANOVA can have one or more categorical IVs. For both PCA and FA, the underlying dimensions (i.e., components or factors) can be viewed as IVs that predict the measured variables. A distinction is sometimes made that for FA the factors are latent IVs, whereas for PCA the IVs are linear combinations of the measured variables. ANCOVA is the only method that will always involve one or more covariates, but MR, MAN(C)OVA, DFA, and LR also may include covariates. CC, PCA, and FA are less likely to include covariates. All the methods involve one or more DVs, with four of them (MR, ANCOVA, DFA, and LR) usually allowing only a single DV. MANOVA and CC allow two or more continuous DVs, and with both PCA and FA we can view the set of two or more measured variables as DVs emanating from the underlying IV dimensions (i.e., components or factors, respectively).

All the methods involve one or more linear combinations. MR forms a linear combination of the IVs, X', that is related to a single, continuous DV. ANCOVA describes the outcome variable, Y, as a linear combination of the grand mean plus a treatment effect and error. MANOVA and DFA each form p or $k - 1$ (whichever is smaller) linear combinations of the continuous variables before examining groups differences. LR forms a single linear combination of the IVs that is related to a single categorical DV. CC forms either p or q (whichever is less) linear combinations on both the IV and DV sides. PCA forms linear combinations of the components (i.e., Vs), whereas FA forms linear combinations of the measured X variables.

Finally, all the methods could involve practical applications based on the results of the analyses. This is especially true for LR that is often applied in medical contexts when the outcome is the presence or absence of a disease, or even death

TABLE 12.1

Multiplicity Themes Applied to Multivariate Methods

	MR	ANCOVA	MANOVA	DFA	LR	CC	PCA	FA
+Theories	Yes	Yes	Yes	Yes	May	May	May	May
+Hypotheses	Yes	May	Yes	Yes	Yes	May	May	May
+Empirical Research	Yes	Yes	Yes	Yes	May	May	May	May
+Time Points	May	May	May	May	May	May	Not Likely	Not Likely
+Controls	May	Yes	May	May	May	May	Not Likely	Not Likely
+Groups	Not Likely	For IV	For IV	For DV	For DV	Not Likely	Not Likely	Not Likely
+IVs	2+	1+	1+	2+	2+	2+	1+	1 + (Latent)
Covariate(s)	May	1+	May	May	May	Not Likely	Not Likely	Not Likely
+DVs	1	1	2+	1	1	2+	2+	2+
+Dimensions	No	No	Yes	Yes	No	Yes	Yes	Yes
+Linear Combos.	1	1	Min (p, k−1)	Min (p, k−1)	1	Min (p, q)	1 + Comps.	2 + Variables
+Pract. Applications	May	May	May	May	Usually	May	May	May

Note: + = multiple, MR = multiple regression, ANCOVA = analysis of covariance, MANOVA = multivariate analysis of variance, DFA = discriminant function analysis, LR = logistic regression, CC = canonical correlation, PCA = principal components analysis, FA = factor analysis, IV = independent variable, DV = dependent variable, Linear Combos = linear combinations, Min = minimum, Comps. = components, Pract. Applications = practical applications.

versus survival of an illness. In these cases, results are sometimes used to assist practitioners with diagnosis or risk assessment for certain diseases.

We now consider background themes for each of the multivariate methods discussed in this book.

WHAT ARE THE MAIN BACKGROUND THEMES APPLIED TO METHODS?

Table 12.2 presents an overview of the background themes applied to the multivariate methods we have covered.

Sample size is not always clear cut but some guidelines can be offered. For prediction methods (e.g., MR, DFA, LR, and CC), we often like to have at least 5 and up to 50 participants per variable with at least 100 or more overall, depending on the nature of the data and the analyses (Green, 1991). With violations of assumptions or stepwise procedures that capitalize on chance variation in the data, more participants are required. For group difference methods (e.g., ANCOVA and MANOVA), a reasonable guideline is to have at least 20 participants per group for each DV. For PCA and FA, a sample size of at least 200 to 400 is usually required (Comrey & Lee, 1992), with larger samples needed (e.g., 400 or more) when many variables are analyzed or when the size of the loadings is only moderate (e.g., | 0.30 to 0.40 |). When loadings are large (e.g., | 0.70 | or higher) and/or there are relatively few measured variables (e.g., 6 to 12), smaller sample sizes (e.g., 100 to 200) may be acceptable to define a stable structure for the underlying dimensions (Guadagnoli & Velicer, 1988).

All the methods tend to involve one or more continuous variables, but LR may be conducted with all categorical variables. Four of the methods (ANCOVA, MANOVA, DFA, and LR) involve one or more categorical variables. All the methods except PCA and FA can include moderator variables that are interactions of two IVs, whereas only three of the methods (MR, ANCVOA, and LR) are likely to include mediators that intervene between IVs and DVs.

The four methods that involve categorical variables (ANCOVA, MANOVA, DFA, and LR) may include descriptive frequencies for the categories or groups. Descriptive means and standard deviations are usually presented for both ANCOVA and MANOVA, but they also may be presented for other methods (MR, DFA, LR, and CC).

The three main assumptions of normality, linearity, and homoscedasticity are usually required for these multivariate methods, except when using a purely descriptive approach (e.g., with some uses of LR, PCA, and FA). The assumption of homogeneity of regression (i.e., equal regressions between the covariate and DV across all levels of the IV) is also required for ANCOVA.

Finally, we often delineate the type of method as prediction (MR, DFA, LR, and sometimes CC), group difference (ANCOVA and MANOVA), or exploratory correlational structure (PCA and FA).

TABLE 12.2
Background Themes Applied to Multivariate Methods

	MR	ANCOVA	MANOVA	DFA	LR	CC	PCA	FA
Sample Size	5–50 per IV	20+ per group	(k)20+ per DV	5–50 per IV	5–50 per IV	5–50 per vble	100–200+	100–200+
Cont Vbles	Usually All	DV & Cov	DVs	IVs	IVs OK	Usually All	Usually All	Usually All
Categ Vbles	Not Likely	Yes for IV(s)	Yes for IV(s)	Yes for DV(s)	Yes for DV	Not Likely	Not Likely	Not Likely
Moderator(s)	May	May	May	May	May	May	Not Likely	Not Likely
Mediator(s)	May	May	Not Likely	Not Likely	May	Not Likely	Not Likely	Not Likely
Descr Freqs	Not Likely	Yes	Yes	Yes	Yes	Not Likely	Not Likely	Not Likely
Means & SDs	May	Yes	Yes	May	May	May	Yes	Yes
Linearity	Yes	Yes	Yes	Yes	May	Yes	Yes	Yes
Normality	Yes	Yes	Yes	Yes	May	Yes	May	May
Homoscedas.	Yes	Yes	Yes	Yes	May	Yes	May	May
Homog. Regr	No	Yes	May	No	No	No	No	No
Method Type	Prediction	Group Diff.	Group Diff.	Prediction	Prediction	Correlation	Corr Structure	Corr Structure

Note: MR = multiple regression, ANCOVA = analysis of covariance, MANOVA = multivariate analysis of variance, DFA = discriminant function analysis, LR = logistic regression, CC = canonical correlation, PCA = principal components analysis, FA = factor analysis, IV = independent variable, k = number of groups, DV = dependent variable, Vble = variable, Cont = continuous, Categ = categorical, Descr Freqs = descriptive frequencies, SDs = standard deviations, Homoscedas. = homoscedasticity, Homog. Regr = homogeneity of regressions, Diff. = differences, Corr Structure = correlational structure.

WHAT ARE THE STATISTICAL MODELS THAT ARE TESTED WITH MULTIVARIATE METHODS?

The statistical models for each multivariate method are presented at the top of Table 12.3. The models, discussed in the chapters, parallel the type of method, whether prediction (MR, DFA, LR), group difference (ANCOVA and MANOVA), correlational (CC), or correlational structure (PCA and FA). Note that most of the methods model the measured (outcome) variables (either Ys, Vs, or Xs) as functions of other variables (e.g., Xs), factors (e.g., F), means, treatment effects, and/or error (i.e., E). CC is unique in modeling the ratio of correlations between variables over the correlations within IVs and DVs.

HOW DO CENTRAL THEMES OF VARIANCE, COVARIANCE, AND LINEAR COMBINATIONS APPLY TO MULTIVARIATE METHODS?

The central themes of variance, covariance, and ratios are outlined in the bottom portion of Table 12.3. In five of the methods (MR, ANCOVA, MANOVA, DFA, and LR), we are interested in the proportion of variance in the DV that is explained by the IVs. For CC, we are interested in the shared variance between pairs of canonical variates, labeled as Vs and Ws that are linear combinations for IVs and DVs, respectively. In both PCA and FA, we are concerned with the variance in the measured variables that is explained by the set of dimensions, labeled components or factors, respectively. For all the methods, we are interested in the covariances among the measures. For both PCA and FA, we may also examine the covariation among dimensions when we use an oblique rotation procedure.

Finally, we are always interested in some ratio of between over within information for the multivariate methods discussed here. The correlational methods of CC, PCA, and FA involve the ratio of covariance between two variables divided by the square root of the product of the respective variances within each variable. For MR, the numerator of the ratio is this same covariance between an X and Y, whereas the denominator is simply the variance within X when forming a regression coefficient. For ANCOVA, we focus on the ratio of between-group variance over within-group variance when performing an F-test. For both MANOVA and DFA, we focus on this same between-group over within-group information, except that the ratio involves matrices and not just single numbers. In LR, we examine odds ratios that give the probability of falling in a reference category (e.g., maintenance stage) with an increase of one point in the IV after taking into account the other variables in the equation.

TABLE 12.3

Models and Central Themes Applied to Multivariate Methods

	MR	ANCOVA	MANOVA	DFA	LR	CC	PCA	FA
Model	$Y = A + BX + \cdots + E$	$Y = \text{Grand } M + \tau + E$	$Y = \text{Grand } M + \tau + E$ and $V = bX + \cdots + bX$	$V = bX + \cdots + bX$	$Y = X' + E$ See X' below	$Rcc = Ryy^{-1}Ryx \ Rxx^{-1}Rxy$	$V = bx + \cdots + bx$	$X = LF + E$
Variance	In DV explained by IVs	In DV explained by IVs	In DVs explained by IVs	In DV explained by IVs	In DVs explained by IVs	In Ws explained by Vs	In measures explained by components	In measures explained by factors
Covariance	Among IVs & DV	Between DV & Covariate	Among DVs	Among IVs	Among Measures	Among Measures	Among Measures & Components	Among Measures & Factors
Ratio	$Cov(x,y)/ \ \sqrt{[\sigma2(x)] \ [\sigma2(x)]}$	BG/WG Variances	$E^{-1}H$	$E^{-1}H$	Odds Ratio	$Cov(x,y)/ \ \sqrt{[\sigma2(x)] \ [\sigma2(y)]}$	$Cov(x,y)/ \ \sqrt{[\sigma2(x)] \ [\sigma2(y)]}$	$Cov(x,y)/ \ \sqrt{[\sigma2(x)] \ [\sigma2(y)]}$

Note: MR = multiple regression, ANCOVA = analysis of covariance, MANOVA = multivariate analysis of variance, DFA = discriminant function analysis, LR = logistic regression, CC = canonical correlation, PCA = principal components analysis, FA = factor analysis, IV = X = independent variable, DV = Y = dependent variable, V = linear combination for X's, W = linear combination for Y's, Cov. = covariance, $[\sigma2(x)]$ = variance of x, BG = between groups, WG = within groups, $E^{-1}H$ = BG variance-covariance hypothesis matrix over WG variance-covariance error matrix, A = intercept, B & b = unstandardized weight, M = mean, τ = treatment effect, E = error, R = correlation matrix, R^{-1} = inverse of a correlation matrix, F = factor, L = factor loading, $X' = [e^{A+B1X1+B2X2+B3X3+B4X4}]/[1 + e^{A+B1X1+B2X2+B3X3+B4X4}]$ for LR.

In the next two sections, we summarize macro- and micro-level assessment for the multivariate methods discussed in this book.

WHAT ARE THE MAIN THEMES NEEDED TO INTERPRET MULTIVARIATE RESULTS AT A MACRO-LEVEL?

Table 12.4 presents an overview of macro-, mid-, and micro-levels of assessment. All the methods, with the usual exception of PCA and FA, rely on a macro-level significance test. Although PCA and FA can use a chi-square-based test of significance to identify the correct number of factors, this test is rarely used (Gorsuch, 1983). Most of the methods (i.e., MR, ANCOVA, MANOVA, DFA, and CC) use an F-test to assess macro-level significance. LR uses a chi-square-based significance test at the macro-level. At the macro-level, all the methods look at some form of shared variance. For MR, ANCOVA, LR, and CC R^2 provides an indication of the macro-level effect size between IVs and DVs. For MANOVA and DFA, the macro-level ES is usually η^2, which is formed from subtracting Wilks's lambda from 1.0. In both PCA and FA, we usually strive to explain at least 50% of the variance in the variables with the set of dimensions that is retained.

Several of the methods involve a mid-level of assessment when interpreting results. With MANOVA, we usually assess which DVs are important by conducting p follow-up ANOVAs (but p ANCOVAs or one DFA could be conducted instead) at the mid-level. In DFA, we examine the significance of the discriminant functions at the mid-level, whereas with CC we examine the squared canonical correlations (i.e., r_c^2) between pairs of canonical variates. For PCA and FA, we verify the number of underlying dimensions at the mid-level, before going on to examine micro-level assessment, discussed next.

WHAT ARE THE MAIN THEMES NEEDED TO INTERPRET MULTIVARIATE RESULTS AT A MICRO-LEVEL?

Some of the methods (MR, ANCOVA, MANOVA, and LR) provide micro-level significance tests (i.e., t-tests, Tukey tests, or Wald tests). All the methods, however, provide some form of micro-level effect size information. For MR, we can examine standardized beta weights [e.g., 0.1, 0.3, and 0.5 for small, medium, and large effect sizes (ESs): Cohen, 1992], or we can square them to interpret as univariate ESs (i.e., 0.01, 0.06, and 0.13 for small, medium, and large ESs). For both ANCOVA and MANOVA, we can calculate Cohen's (1988) d to assess the importance of the mean differences (with values of 0.2, 0.5, and 0.8 representing small, medium, and large univariate ESs). DFA, CC, PCA, and FA focus on loadings that are at least

TABLE 12.4
Interpretation Themes Applied to Multivariate Methods

	MR	ANCOVA	MANOVA	DFA	LR	CC	PCA	FA
Macro-Fit Significance Test	F	F	F	F	χ^2	F	(Usually none)	(Usually none)
Macro-Fit Effect Size	R^2 with .02, .13 & .26 for small to large	R^2 with .02, .13 & .26 for small to large	η^2 with .02, .13 & .26 for small to large	η^2 with .02, .13 & .26 for small to large	R^2 with .02, .13 & .26 for small to large	R^2 with .02, .13 & .26 for small to large	≥50% of X's explained variance	≥50% of X's explained variance
Mid-Level Assessment			ANOVAs	Discriminant functions		r_c^2 between canonical variate pairs	Number of factors	Number of components
Micro-Level Significance Test	t-test p < .05 or p < .01	Tukey tests p < .05 or p < .01	Tukey tests p < .05 or p < .01		Wald tests p < .05 or p < .01			
Micro-Level Effect Size	Beta weights .1, .3 & .5 for small to large	Cohen's d .2, .5 & .8 for small to large	Cohen's d .2, .5 & .8 for small to large	Discriminant loadings >|.30|	Odds ratios >1 or <1 are preferred	Canonical loadings >|.30|	Loadings >|.30|	Loadings >|.30|

Note: IV = independent variable, DV = dependent variable, Cov. = covariance, MR = multiple regression, ANCOVA = analysis of covariance, MANOVA = multivariate analysis of variance, DFA = discriminant function analysis, LR = logistic regression, CC = canonical correlation, PCA = principal components analysis, FA = factor analysis, ANOVAs, analyses of variance, $R^2 = \eta^2$ = percent of shared variance between Xs and Ys.

| 0.30 | at the micro-level, also allowing squared values that can be interpreted as small, medium, and large ESs for values of 0.01, 0.06, and 0.13, respectively.

WHAT ARE SOME OTHER CONSIDERATIONS OR NEXT STEPS AFTER APPLYING MULTIVARIATE METHODS?

After conducting any multivariate method, it is important to consider possible future steps that would illuminate or verify the current findings. The ultimate goal is to be able to find reliable and valid results that generalize beyond a specific sample. Often it is useful to replicate findings, possibly with different kinds of samples, measures, or methods. If similar results occur, there is much greater verisimilitude in the findings.

WHAT ARE EXAMPLES OF APPLYING MULTIVARIATE METHODS TO RELEVANT RESEARCH QUESTIONS?

Throughout this book, we have examined applications on a single data set (see accompanying CD) collected from 527 women at risk for HIV. Each of the examples relied on the theoretical frameworks of the transtheoretical model (Prochaska et al., 1994a, 1994b) and the multifaceted model of HIV risk (Harlow et al., 1993, 1998). In most of the examples (for MR, MANOVA, DFA, and LR), we analyzed the relationships between psychosexual functioning, the pros and cons of condom use, and condom self-efficacy, on the one hand, and stages of condom use on the other hand. For ANCOVA, we examined the cons of condom use at the initial time point as a covariate, with the second time point providing data for the DV. As with the MANOVA example, the five stages of condom use (1, precontemplation; 2, contemplation; 3, preparation; 4, action; and 5, maintenance) served as levels of the IV. For CC, we analyzed the relationship among all five variables (psychosexual functioning, pros, cons, condom self-efficacy, and stage of condom use) at two different time points, collected 6 months apart.

Analyses from each of these applications showed that there was significant shared variance among the variables, particularly with condom self-efficacy and stages of condom use, with psychosexual functioning having less in common with stages, and the pros and cons falling somewhere in between.

For PCA and FA, we analyzed three transtheoretical model variables (pros, cons, and condom self-efficacy) with five multifaceted model of HIV risk variables (psychosexual functioning, meaninglessness, stress, demoralization, and powerlessness). These analyses resulted in two dimensions (i.e., for the trans-theoretical model and multifaceted model of HIV risk variables, respectively) to explain the pattern of correlations among the variables.

It is hoped that the presentation of various themes that cut across all the methods, with theoretically anchored applications for each method, provided a useful framework for understanding the essence of multivariate methods. It is up to the imagination and energy of the reader to further explore how to apply these methods to a wide range of phenomena, generating far-reaching implications and a strong knowledge base in the fields in which the multivariate methods are applied.

REFERENCES

Cohen, J. (1988). *Statistical power analysis for the behavioral sciences.* San Diego, CA: Academic Press.

Cohen, J. (1992). A power primer. *Psychological Bulletin, 112*, 155–159.

Comrey, A. L., & Lee, H. B. (1992). *A first course in factor analysis* (2nd ed.). Hillsdale, NJ: Lawrence Erlbaum Associates.

Gorsuch, R. L. (1983). *Factor Analysis* (2nd ed.). Hillsdale, NJ: Erlbaum.

Green, S. B. (1991). How many subjects does it take to do a regression analysis? *Multivariate Behavioral Research, 26*, 449–510.

Guadagnoli, E., & Velicer, W. F. (1988). Relation of sample size to the stability of component patterns. *Psychological Bulletin, 10*, 265–275.

Harlow, L. L., Quina, K., Morokoff, P. J., Rose, J. S., & Grimley, D. (1993). HIV risk in women: A multifaceted model. *Journal of Applied Biobehavioral Research, 1*, 3–38.

Harlow, L., Rose, J., Morokoff, P., Quina, K., Mayer, K., Mitchell, K., & Schnoll, R. (1998). Women HIV sexual risk takers: Related behaviors, interpersonal issues & attitudes. *Women's Health: Research on Gender, Behavior and Policy, 4*, 407–439.

Prochaska, J. O., Redding, C. A., Harlow, L. L., Rossi, J. S., & Velicer, W. F. (1994a). The Transtheoretical model and HIV prevention: A review. *Health Education Quarterly, 21*, 45–60.

Prochaska, J. O., Velicer, W. F., Rossi, J. S., Goldstein, M. G., Marcus, B. H., Rakowski, W., Fiore, C., Harlow, L. L., Redding, C. A., Rosenbloom, D., & Rossi, S. R. (1994b). Stages of change and decisional balance for 12 problem behaviors. *Health Psychology, 13*, 39–46.

Author Index

Note: Numbers in *italics* indicate pages with complete bibliographic information.

A

Abelson, R. P., 5, 6, *8*, 11, 12, *25*
Aiken, L. S., 4, *9*, 16, 23, 24, *26*, 33, 35, *39*, 44, 45, 46, 47, 59, *61*, 177, *197*
Aldrich, J. H., 154, *173*
Allison, P. D., 33, *39*
Alsup, R., 30, *39*
Alwin, D. F., 15, *25*
Anastasi, A., 12, *25*
Anderson, R. E., 65, *80*
APA Task Force on Statistical Inference, 6, *9*, 21, 22, *27*

B

Baron, R. M., 30, *39*
Bentler, P. M., 6, *8*, 15, *25*, 208, *216*
Berkson, J., 5, *8*
Black, W. C., 65, *80*
Bock, R. D., 114, *127*
Boomsma, A., 6, *8*
Brandt, U., 30, *40*
Britt, D. W., 37, *39*
Browne, M. W., 14, *26*
Bullock, H. E., 13, *25*
Byrne, B. M., 30, *39*, 208, *216*

C

Campbell, D. T., 14, *27*
Campbell, K. T., 177, *197*
Carmer, S. G., 24, *25*
Cattell, R. B., 206, 210, *216*
Chassin, L., 152, *173*
Cohen, J., 4, 6, *9*, 16, 22, 23, 24, *25*, *26*, 33, 35, *39*, 44, 45, 46, 47, 48, 59, *61*, 67, 71, 74, *80*, 108, 109, 113, 115, *127*, 134, 136, *150*, 157, 161, 165, *173*, 177, 181, *197*, 229, 230, *232*
Cohen, P., 4, *9*, 16, 23, 24, *26*, 33, 35, *39*, 44, 45, 46, 47, 59, *61*, 177, *197*
Collins, L. M., 13, *26*, 30, 33, *39*
Collyer, C. E., 14, *26*
Comrey, A. L., 7, *9*, 202, *216*, 225, *232*
Cook, T. D., 14, *27*
Cudeck, R., 14, *26*

D

Delaney, H. D., 15, *26*
Devlin, K., 28, 37, *39*
Diener, E., 15, *26*
Dwyer, J. H., 30, *40*

233

Subject Index